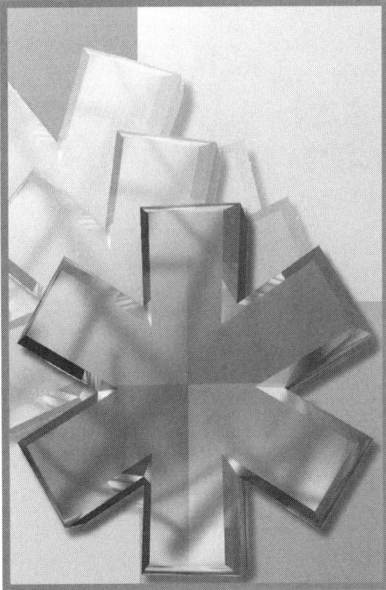

BRADY

ADVANCED MEDICAL LIFE SUPPORT

A PRACTICAL APPROACH TO ADULT MEDICAL EMERGENCIES

THIRD EDITION

Coordinator & Instructor Guide

Linda M. Abrahamson, BA, RN, EMT-P
EMS Education Coordinator, Silver Cross Hospital/Joliet Junior College, Joliet, Illinois

Rosemary Adam, RN, EMT-P
Emergency Medicine Educator/Nurse Instructor, The University of Iowa Health Care
EMS Learning Resources Center, Iowa City, Iowa

Ann Bellows, RN, EMT-P, Ed.D.
Training Coordinator, Southwest Air Ambulance, Las Cruces, New Mexico

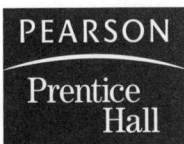
PEARSON
Prentice
Hall

Upper Saddle River, New Jersey 07458

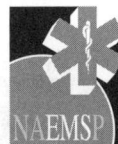
NAEMSP

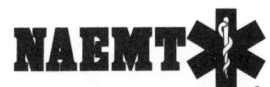
NAEMT

Publisher: *Julie Levin Alexander*
Publisher's Assistant: *Regina Bruno*
Senior Acquisitions Editor: *Stephen Smith*
Senior Managing Editor for Development: *Lois Berlowitz*
Project Manager: *Sandy Breuer*
Editorial Assistant: *Diane Edwards*
Associate Editor: *Monica Moosang*
Director of Marketing: *Karen Allman*
Executive Marketing Manager: *Katrin Beacom*
Marketing Coordinator: *Michael Sirinides*
Marketing Assistant: *Wayne Celia, Jr.*
Managing Production Editor: *Patrick Walsh*
Production Liaison: *Julie Li*
Production Editor: *Peggy Hood, Techbooks*
Media Product Manager: *John Jordan*
Manager of Media Production: *Amy Peltier*
New Media Project Manager: *Tina Rudowski*
Manufacturing Manager: *Ilene Sanford*
Manufacturing Buyer: *Pat Brown*
Senior Design Coordinator: *Christopher Weigand*
Composition: *Techbooks*
Printing and Binding: *Bind Rite Graphics*
Cover Printer: *Phoenix Color Corporation*

This book was set in 11/13 Times by *Techbooks*. It was printed and bound by Command Web. The cover was printed by Phoenix Color Corporation.

Pearson Education Ltd.
Pearson Education Singapore Pte. Ltd.
Pearson Education Canada, Ltd.
Pearson Education—Japan

Pearson Education Australia Pty. Limited
Pearson Education North Asia Ltd.
Pearson Educación de Mexico, S.A. de C.V.
Pearson Education Malaysia Pte. Ltd.

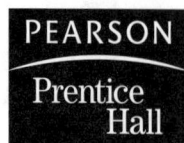

PEARSON
Prentice
Hall

10 9 8 7 6 5 4 3 2 1
ISBN: 0-13-188900-1

DEDICATION

The Advanced Medical Life Support (AMLS) Executive Committee would like to dedicate this edition of the AMLS *Coordinator & Instructor Guide* to all of the AMLS faculty and the patients they cared for whose lives were forever changed because of the aftermath of the 2005 hurricane, Katrina. Our sincere gratitude for your perseverance and dedication to the EMS communities that you serve.

CONTENTS

ABOUT THE AUTHORS

Linda M. Abrahamson, BA, RN, EMT-P, is the EMS education coordinator at Silver Cross Hospital, Joliet, Illinois. She currently manages a community college paramedic program and continuing education courses for a multi-county EMS System. She is a flight paramedic and emergency room registered nurse. Linda has served many local and national EMS leadership roles in national EMS organizations. She is the past president of the National Association of EMS Educators (NAEMSE). She is the chairperson for the National Association of Emergency Medical Technicians (NAEMT) Advanced Medical Life Support Executive Committee.

Rosemary Adam, RN, EMT-P, is an EMS nurse, flight nurse, and emergency medicine educator with 25 years of experience. She has been active in Iowa and the Midwest in the design, development, coordination, and presentation of many different types of educational programs for EMS providers, nurses, and physicians.

Ann Bellows, RN, EMT-P, Ed.D., is the training coordinator for Southwest Air Ambulance, Las Cruces, New Mexico. She has over 20 years of experience in prehospital education. She has worked in intensive care units (ICUs) and emergency departments (EDs) in small rural hospitals and Level I Trauma Centers. She has clinical experience in fixed and rotor-wing transport. She is involved with the NAEMT and has worked to develop the pre-hospital trauma life support (PHTLS) and AMLS courses. Ann has been the program coordinator and primary instructor for EMS classes at all levels. She has her doctorate in training and learning technologies with a minor in message design.

ACKNOWLEDGMENTS

The authors wish to acknowledge and thank the following contributors to the third edition of this *Coordinator & Instructor Guide*. Their contributions to developing a more internationally accepted instructor tool and standardizing NAEMT policies within the *Guide* were invaluable.

Vincent N. Mosesso, Jr., MD
University of Pittsburgh
Emergency Medicine
Pittsburgh, PA

Keshia Robinson
NAEMT AMLS Coordinator
Clinton, MS

John Greg Clarkes, NREMT-P
President/Education Coordinator
Canadian College of EMS
Edmonton, Alberta, Canada

The AMLS Executive Committee commends our International AMLS Sites for their support of NAEMT and their vision and commitment to quality patient care. To date, the following countries have implemented AMLS as a patient care standard:

Argentina	Hong Kong	Switzerland
Canada	Italy	Trinidad/Tobago
Columbia	Norway	United Kingdom

ADVANCED MEDICAL LIFE SUPPORT
EXECUTIVE COMMITTEE

Linda M. Abrahamson, BA, RN, EMT-P
AMLS Chairperson
EMS Education Coordinator
Silver Cross Hospital/Joliet Junior
  College
Joliet, IL

Vincent N. Mosesso, Jr., MD
National Association of Emergency
  Medical Services Physicians
  (NAEMSP)
AMLS Medical Director
University of Pittsburgh Emergency
  Medicine
Pittsburgh, PA

**Rosemary Adam, RN, EMT-P
(Specialist)**
Nurse Instructor
The University of Iowa Health Care
  EMS Learning Resources Center
Iowa City, IA

Ann Bellows, RN, EMT-P, Ed.D.
Training Coordinator
Southwest Air Ambulance
Las Cruces, NM

**John Greg Clarkes, EMT-P,
  MICP, NREMT-P**
President and Education Coordinator
Canadian College of EMS
Edmonton General Hospital
Edmonton, Alberta, Canada

Will Chapleau, RN, EMT-P
Chief
Chicago Heights Fire Department
Chicago Heights, IL

FOREWORD

In 1984, I presented a two-day course on the management of adult medical emergencies to fifty physicians and nurses in Havre, Montana. Based on the already-existing model of "Advanced Cardiac Life Support" and "Advanced Trauma Life Support," the course was named "Advanced Medical Life Support" or "AMLS" for short. Over the next several years, numerous nurses, physicians, EMTs, and paramedics participated in this course. In 1987, my text *Advanced Medical Life Support—Adult Medical Emergencies* was published. Despite initial interest, the time may not have been right, for interest in the course and the text waned. And, my efforts moved in other directions.

The need for a nationally based and standardized course on the treatment of adult medical emergencies, especially to out-of-hospital personnel, has not changed. Today, through the efforts of both NAEMSP and NAEMT, this concept has become a reality. While Twink, Dan, Joe, and Howie have written the AMLS textbook, an NAEMT Course Committee has formulated and will promote the AMLS course. Both the textbook and course are aimed directly at paramedics and employ time-tested strategies. Though I was not personally involved, I derive great satisfaction from seeing the AMLS concept take shape on a large scale. With all the current changes in national EMS, the time seems ripe.

I wish all involved my best.

Mikel A. Rothenberg, MD
Emergency Care Educator
North Olmsted, OH

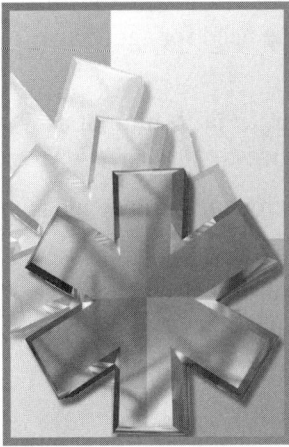

I. PROVIDER COURSE OBJECTIVES

ASSESSMENT OF THE MEDICAL PATIENT

Given a scenario, the participant will be able to apply critical thinking skills to integrate pathophysiology with assessment and history findings to determine actual and potential patient problems, differential diagnoses, and management strategies.

KEYS *The participant will be able to:*

1) Demonstrate with proficiency an appropriate, safe scene size-up.

2) Differentiate treatment and transport criteria for stable and unstable patients.

3) Differentiate appropriate assessment techniques for stable and unstable adult patients with medical complaints.

4) Obtain a comprehensive patient assessment using appropriate interviewing techniques.

5) Recognize and explain different pathophysiological responses found during the comprehensive assessment of patients with medical complaints.

6) Describe the rationale for assessment modifications used for the elderly patient.

7) Demonstrate an efficient, focused physical examination technique for evaluating patients with neurological, respiratory, cardiac, and abdominal complaints.

AIRWAY MANAGEMENT, VENTILATION, AND OXYGEN THERAPY

Given a scenario, the participant will be able to apply critical thinking skills to integrate pathophysiology with assessment and history findings to determine actual and potential patient problems, differential diagnoses, and management strategies.

KEYS *The participant will be able to:*

1) Demonstrate with proficiency an appropriate, safe scene size-up.

2) Recognize patient presentations that require the need for aggressive airway management.

3) Identify different clinical situations that determine utilization of a variety of options for airway management devices.

4) Explain the indications and contra-indications for each airway management technique or device.

5) Demonstrate with proficiency the appropriate use of airway management techniques that include:

   a) Oral tracheal intubation

   b) Nasal tracheal intubation

   c) Rapid sequence intubation

   d) Digital intubation

   e) Lighted-stylet intubation

   f) Alternative airway devices (PtL®, Combitube®, LMA®)

   g) Surgical airway alternatives

⊞ HYPOPERFUSION (SHOCK)

Given a scenario, the participant will be able to apply critical thinking skills to integrate pathophysiology with assessment and history findings to determine actual and potential patient problems, differential diagnoses, and management strategies.

KEYS *The participant will be able to:*

1) Demonstrate with proficiency an appropriate, safe scene size-up.

2) Identify differences in patient presentations in compensated, progressive, and irreversible shock.

3) Use, with proficiency, a comprehensive assessment technique to identify differences in patient presentations and management strategies for hypovolemic, obstructive, distributive, and cardiogenic shock.

4) Recognize and explain different pathophysiological responses found during the comprehensive assessment of patients exhibiting hypovolemic, obstructive, distributive, and cardiogenic shock.

5) Develop management alternatives for probable differential diagnoses of hypoperfusion to include as needed: airway management, respiratory and/or ventilatory support, fluid therapy, pharmacological support, and transportation to an appropriate facility.

⊞ DYSPNEA

Given a scenario, the participant will be able to apply critical thinking skills to integrate pathophysiology with assessment and history findings to determine actual and potential patient problems, differential diagnoses, and management strategies.

KEYS *The participant will be able to:*

1) Demonstrate with proficiency an appropriate, safe scene size-up.

2) Identify differences in patient presentation and management strategies for patients that exhibit respiratory distress and respiratory failure.

3) Recognize and explain with accuracy different pathophysiological responses found during the comprehensive assessment of patients exhibiting airway obstruction, asthma, chronic obstructive pulmonary disorder (COPD), pneumonia, pleural effusion, tension pneumothorax, pulmonary embolism, pleuritis, adult respiratory distress syndrome (ARDS), congestive heart failure (CHF), acute myocardial infarction (AMI), neuromuscular dystrophies, hyperthyroidism, and psychogenic etiologies.

4) Use a comprehensive assessment technique to identify differences in patient presentations and management strategies for airway obstruction, asthma, COPD, pneumonia, pleural effusion, tension pneumothorax, pulmonary embolus, pleuritis, ARDS, CHF, AMI, neuromuscular dystrophies, hyperthyroidism, and psychogenic etiologies.

5) Develop management alternatives for probable differential diagnoses of dyspnea to include as needed: airway management, respiratory and/or ventilatory support, fluid therapy, pharmacological support, and transportation to an appropriate facility.

CHEST PAIN

Given a scenario, the participant will be able to apply critical thinking skills to integrate pathophysiology with assessment and history findings to determine actual and potential patient problems, differential diagnosis, and management stratagies.

KEYS *The participant will be able to:*

1) Demonstrate with proficiency an appropriate, safe scene size-up.

2) Identify differences in patient presentation and management strategies for patients that exhibit AMI, unstable angina, aortic dissection, pulmonary embolism, esophageal disruption, cardiac tamponade, pericarditis, costochondritis, gastrointestinal disease, and mitral valve prolapse.

3) Recognize and explain with accuracy different pathophysiological responses found during the comprehensive assessment of patients exhibiting AMI, unstable angina, aortic dissection, pulmonary embolism, esophageal disruption, cardiac tamponade, pericarditis, costochondritis, gastrointestinal disease, and mitral valve prolapse.

4) Develop management alternatives for probable differential diagnoses of chest pain to include as needed: airway management, respiratory and/or ventilatory support, fluid therapy, pharmacological support, and transportation to an appropriate facility.

⊞ ALTERED MENTAL STATUS

Given a scenario, the participant will be able to apply critical thinking skills to integrate pathophysiology with assessment and history findings to determine actual and potential patient problems, differential diagnosis, and management strategies.

KEYS *The participant will be able to:*

1) Demonstrate with proficiency an appropriate, safe scene size-up.

2) Identify differences in patient presentation and management strategies for patients that exhibit a cerebral vascular accident (CVA), transient ischemic attack (TIA), cranial infections, intracranial tumors, diabetes mellitus, hyperglycemic hyperosmolar nonketotic syndrome, hepatic encephalopathy, uremic encephalopathy, electrolyte imbalances, acidosis and alkalosis, thyroid disorders, Wernicke's encephalopathy, Korsakoff's psychosis, toxicologic encephalopathy, and environmental etiologies.

3) Recognize and explain with accuracy different pathophysiological responses found during the comprehensive assessment of patients exhibiting CVA, TIA, cranial infections, intracranial tumors, diabetes mellitus, hyperglycemic hyperosmolar nonketotic syndrome, hepatic encephalopathy, uremic encephalopathy, electrolyte imbalances, acidosis and alkalosis, thyroid disorders, Wernicke's encephalopathy, Korsakoff's psychosis, toxicologic encephalopathy, and environmental etiologies.

4) Develop management alternatives for probable differential diagnoses of altered mental status to include as needed: airway management, respiratory and/or ventilatory support, fluid therapy, pharmacological support, and transportation to an appropriate facility.

⊞ SEIZURES AND SEIZURE DISORDERS

Given a scenario, the participant will be able to apply critical thinking skills to integrate pathophysiology with assessment and history findings to determine actual and potential patient problems, differential diagnosis, and management strategies.

KEYS *The participant will be able to:*

1) Demonstrate with proficiency an appropriate, safe scene size-up.

2) Identify differences in patient presentation and management strategies for patients that exhibit generalized, simple or partial complex seizures, status epilepticus, metabolic disorders, and infectious diseases.

3) Recognize and explain with accuracy different pathophysiological responses found during the comprehensive assessment of patients exhibiting generalized, simple or partial complex seizures, status epilepticus, metabolic disorders, and infectious diseases.

4) Develop management alternatives for probable differential diagnoses of seizures to include as needed: airway management, respiratory and/or ventilatory support, fluid therapy, pharmacological support, and transportation to an appropriate facility.

ACUTE ABDOMINAL PAIN/GI BLEEDING

Given a scenario, the participant will be able to apply critical thinking skills to integrate pathophysiology with assessment and history findings to determine actual and potential patient problems, differential diagnosis, and management strategies.

KEYS *The participant will be able to:*

1) Demonstrate with proficiency an appropriate, safe scene size-up.

2) Identify differences in patient presentation and management strategies for patients that exhibit right and left hypochondriac, epigastric, umbilical, hypogastric, aortic aneurysm, gastric-esophageal reflux disease (GERD), and right and left iliac region etiologies.

3) Recognize and explain with accuracy different pathophysiological responses found during the comprehensive assessment of patients exhibiting right and left hypochondriac, epigastric, umbilical, hypogastric, aortic aneurysm, GERD, and right and left iliac region etiologies.

4) Identify anatomical locations that are at risk for gastrointestinal bleeding.

5) Recognize and explain with accuracy different pathophysiological responses found during the comprehensive assessment of patients exhibiting presentations and predisposing conditions to gastrointestinal bleeding.

6) Develop management alternatives for probable differential diagnoses of acute abdominal pain and gastrointestinal bleeding to include as needed: airway management, respiratory and/or ventilatory support, fluid therapy, pharmacological support, and transportation to an appropriate facility.

SYNCOPE

Given a scenario, the participant will be able to apply critical thinking skills to integrate pathophysiology with assessment and history findings to determine actual and potential patient problems, differential diagnosis, and management strategies.

KEYS *The participant will be able to:*

1) Demonstrate with proficiency an appropriate, safe scene size-up.

2) Identify differences in patient presentation and management strategies for patients that exhibit vasovagal and vasopressor syncope, orthostatic hypotension, and metabolic and neurologic syncope etiologies.

3) Recognize and explain with accuracy different pathophysiological responses found during the comprehensive assessment of patients exhibiting vasovagal and vasopressor syncope, orthostatic hypotension, and metabolic and neurologic syncope etiologies.

4) Develop management alternatives for probable differential diagnoses of syncope to include as needed: airway management, respiratory and/or ventilatory support, fluid therapy, pharmacological support, and transportation to an appropriate facility.

▦ HEADACHE, NAUSEA, AND VOMITING

Given a scenario, the participant will be able to apply critical thinking skills to integrate pathophysiology with assessment and history findings to determine actual and potential patient problems, differential diagnosis, and management strategies.

KEYS *The participant will be able to:*

1) Demonstrate with proficiency an appropriate, safe scene size-up.

2) Identify differences in patient presentation and management strategies for patients that exhibit tension headaches, migraine, subarachnoid and intracerebral hemorrhage, subdural hematoma, meningitis, pre-eclampsia, carbon monoxide poisoning, and brain abscess, nausea, and vomiting etiologies.

3) Recognize and explain with accuracy different pathophysiological responses found during the comprehensive assessment of patients exhibiting tension headaches, migraine, subarachnoid and intracerebral hemorrhage, subdural hematoma, meningitis, pre-eclampsia, carbon monoxide poisoning, and brain abscess, nausea, and vomiting etiologies.

4) Develop management alternatives for probable differential diagnoses of headache, nausea, and vomiting to include as needed: airway management, respiratory and/or ventilatory support, fluid therapy, pharmacological support, and transportation to an appropriate facility.

▦ INSTRUCTOR COURSE OBJECTIVES

At the conclusion of the instructor course, the instructor candidate will be able to:

1) Describe the correlation between a healthcare practioner's scope of practice and experience and his or her challenges in a classroom setting.

2) Identify the process of course registration using NAEMT educational software.

3) Describe the responsibilities of an AMLS instructor, affiliate faculty, and course coordinator.

4) Identify the purpose of the instructional components in the *AMLS Coordinator & Instructor Guide.*

⊞ REFRESHER COURSE OBJECTIVES

At the conclusion of the refresher course, participants will be able to:

1) Identify with proficiency the components of the AMLS assessment process for adults with various medical complaints.

2) Describe with accuracy the assessment, differential diagnosis, and management of adult patient presentations of difficulties in airway maintenance, dyspnea, chest pain, hypoperfusion, altered mental status, and abdominal pain.

3) Demonstrate with proficiency critical thinking skills that foster the progress of using an assessment-based process during the initial impression assessment and progressing to a diagnoses-based assessment to appropriately manage adult medical complaints.

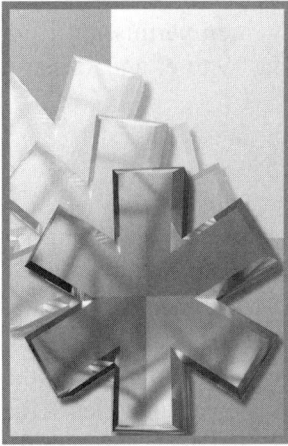

II. ADVANCED MEDICAL LIFE SUPPORT COURSE ADMINISTRATION

NOTES

AMLS MISSION STATEMENT

The mission of the Advanced Medical Life Support (AMLS) program is to promote competence of healthcare providers in the assessment and management of adult patients who experience medical emergencies. The AMLS mission complements the mission of the National Association of Emergency Medical Technicians by providing a quality educational experience through Provider, Instructor, and Refresher programs that enhance the knowledge and skills of healthcare providers. To that end, AMLS provides healthcare providers the opportunity to participate in scenario-based, interactive presentations and hands-on experiences that use comprehensive assessment and history-taking skills, focused physical examinations, and formulation and progression from an initial or field impression to differential diagnoses and appropriate management.

The National Association of Emergency Medical Technicians

The mission of the National Association of Emergency Medical Technicians (NAEMT) is to represent and serve Emergency Medical Services personnel through advocacy, educational programs, and research. NAEMT serves its professional membership through a variety of liaison activities that promote Emergency Medical Services as a recognized allied health profession, The AMLS program is but one of the educational programs offered by the NAEMT.

THE AMLS PROGRAM

Purpose of the *AMLS Coordinator & Instructor Guide,* 3rd Edition

The purpose of this *AMLS Coordinator & Instructor Guide* is to serve as a resource for AMLS instructors and course coordinators. This tool is **required for use** as a companion document to the AMLS textbook when teaching AMLS Provider, Refresher, and Instructor courses. This instructor resource provides the core AMLS course content and ensures consistency within domestic, U.S. military, and international courses.

This document will define NAEMT and AMLS Executive Committee policies and procedures relative to the administration of AMLS Provider, Refresher, and

9

Instructor courses. Course coordinators must obtain written permission from NAEMT to deviate from the prescribed course agenda, lecture, and scenario content.

The AMLS Executive Committee

The group of healthcare professionals and exemplary educators that comprise the AMLS Executive Committee are appointed by the president of NAEMT and function under the auspices of the NAEMT. The AMLS medical director, approved by the NAEMT president, is a representative of the National Association of EMS Physicians (NAEMSP) and ensures that the content within the courses is sound medical practice. Committee members are accountable for the administration and quality of the Provider, Refresher, and Instructor course content. The committee oversees all AMLS domestic, U.S. military, and international faculty.

AMLS Executive Committee Meetings The AMLS Executive Committee meets on a regular basis via conference call and face-to-face meetings. The annual meeting, open to all interested parties, is held in conjunction with the NAEMT annual meeting. AMLS instructors, course coordinators, affiliate/state, military, and provincial/international faculty are encouraged to contact committee members to provide input on AMLS business.

AMLS International Office

The international office is located at 132A East Northside Drive, Clinton, MS 39056. The mailing address is P.O. Box 1400, Clinton, MS 39060-1400. Office personnel can be contacted at 1-800-34-NAEMT (1-800-346-2368).

AMLS Website

The AMLS website can be viewed at http://www.amls.org/. The website posts nationwide and international course information. The website serves AMLS faculty and those seeking information on AMLS.

AMLS faculty may contribute articles or photographs to the website. All contributions should be sent to http://www.amls@naemt.org. All photographs must be accompanied by a signed release by the participants.

AMLS Awards

The AMLS Executive Committee may nominate an AMLS recognized instructor, course coordinator, affiliate/state, or international faculty to be recognized for their contributions to the AMLS mission. This award is presented at the NAEMT annual meeting.

AMLS Logo Usage

Use of the AMLS logo is prohibited without the written consent of the NAEMT. Requests to use the logo for course promotional purposes must be submitted in writing to NAEMT. If approval is granted, written approval will be sent as confirmation. The use of the AMLS logo is encouraged for promotional purposes. The AMLS logo cannot be amended or altered.

International AMLS

The AMLS Executive Committee is committed to working closely with our international colleagues on implementing scenarios and lecture content that is relevant to their culture. International AMLS affiliate faculty and instructors are encouraged to forward recommendations to meet this objective to the AMLS Executive Committee on an ongoing basis.

The AMLS Executive Committee is proud to welcome our international colleagues who have adopted the AMLS philosophy and course for their healthcare providers. At the time of this publication, the following countries have incorporated AMLS into their healthcare continuing education: Argentina, Canada, Columbia, Hong Kong, Italy, Norway, Switzerland, Trinidad/Tobago, and United Kingdom.

Prior to the introduction of AMLS outside the United States, several requirements must be met. An on-site medical director and a core of AMLS instructors must be established prior to the inaugural course. It is preferred that the international site locations have an active pre-hospital trauma life support (PHTLS) site or any other endorsed NAEMT program actively functioning.

It is also preferred that the potential instructors, course coordinators, affiliate faculty, and medical directors travel to the United States and attend an AMLS Provider and Instructor course. The international AMLS courses must be held at a site approved by the AMLS chairperson. This process will ensure the sponsors obtain insight on how the courses are organized.

Once a potential host country has recognized AMLS instructor-candidates, dates are set for the country's inaugural AMLS course. Typically a 2-day Provider and Instructor course and a subsequent 2-day Provider course are scheduled. Participants for the Provider/Instructor courses are selected by the host country. There is typically a 1-day break between the scheduled Provider courses. This break provides an opportunity for the instructor-candidates identified in the inaugural course time to prepare to be monitored and participate as instructors in the second Provider course. The AMLS chairperson or their designee and the AMLS medical director will participate in the inaugural course. They will serve as NAEMT ambassadors and as a resource for the AMLS course philosophy and content. This AMLS leadership serves as affiliate faculty and monitors the instructor-candidates in both courses. International affiliate faculty will be appointed at the inaugural course by the AMLS chairperson or designee present at the inaugural course.

Once course dates have been determined, the president of NAEMT will begin the process for obtaining the signatures on the Memorandum of Understanding (MOU). This MOU is an agreement for maintaining the integrity of the courses and course coordination activities for inaugural and pending courses. The president of NAEMT, the chairperson of the AMLS Executive Committee, the AMLS medical director, and the course director at the international institution hosting the inaugural course will sign the MOU. The conditions outlined in the MOU are strongly adhered to as the inaugural and future courses are established within a country.

Prior approval by the AMLS chairperson is required for international course coordinators to alter the lecture or scenario content of the courses to be appropriate and relevant to local customs and protocols.

Military AMLS Courses

The NAEMT and AMLS Executive Committees support and encourage implementation of the AMLS courses in all branches of the military healthcare provider continuing education.

A surcharge per participant for all AMLS military courses is $10/participant. Military course coordinators will use the NAEMT course software to complete course applications and submit post-course paperwork.

Scenario locations may be adapted to appropriate military environments, but the signs/symptoms and differential diagnoses must remain as indicated in this Guide.

Goals of the Courses

The hands-on portion of each AMLS course gives each participant the ability to integrate the knowledge presented into a practical format for use in his or her current practice. Although the courses strongly emphasize the prehospital management of medical emergencies, each scenario and hands-on practical lab station is easily altered for relevance within scopes of practice for registered nurses, respiratory therapists, physicians, residents, physician assistants, nurse practicioners, nurse anesthesiologists, and other advanced-level healthcare providers. The format and administrative policies set forth are those of the NAEMT.

The major goals of an AMLS course are to:

▶ Apply critical thinking skills in order to integrate pathophysiology with the patient presentation and assessment findings of a medical patient.

   ▶ Determine and differentiate between actual and potential patient diagnoses.

   ▶ Advance the provider's ability to conduct a comprehensive medical examination that uses proper diagnostic, critical thinking, and treatment modality skills.

   ▶ Use problem-solving strategies in interventions and management alternatives.

▶ Allow the participant to systematically work through a patient assessment and examine the possibilities and probabilities of differential diagnoses.

▦ PROVIDER COURSE

Course Philosophy

The Advanced Medical Life Support (AMLS) Provider course is a 2-day (16-hour) in-depth study of medical emergencies for the adult patient. The Provider course emphasizes a pragmatic approach and systematic format regarding patient assessment and management. The course is designed to combine interactive scenario-based lectures with hands-on physical assessments of patients. The participant will practice a global and initial assessment, taking into account the patient's environmental and scene issues. This information will help the participant to formulate a general impression, determine the patient's stability, and explore the possibilities of differential diagnoses. Using a systematic approach to obtain an initial assessment, vital signs, present illness and past medical history, and a focused physical exam, the participant will begin to develop a rationale for probable differential diagnoses. The management of the patient will be driven by the differential diagnoses.

Pre-course preparation is necessary for successful completion of the course. Participants must purchase a current copy of the *Advanced Medical Life Support* textbook and review the pre-course materials. The pre-test must be completed prior to the first day of class.

Successful completion of the program consists of the following:

▶ Attendance at both days of the course

▶ A score of 76% or better on the written final evaluation

▶ Proficiency at the four assessment evaluation stations:

— Dyspnea/Respiratory/Failure, Chest Pain (also includes Hypoperfusion), Abdominal Pain/GI Bleeding, and Altered Mental Status.

Upon successful completion of the competencies in the Provider, Refresher, and Instructor courses, the participant will receive an official AMLS certificate and card. Course coordinators and/or affiliate faculty will award the certificates on the same day as the completion of the course.

Continuing Education Credit

Upon successful completion, the basic and advanced participants will receive 16 hours of continuing education and be awarded an Advanced Medical Life Support Provider certificate and wallet card. The continuing education credits are nationally approved by the NAEMT organizational accreditation by the Continuing Education Coordinating Board of Emergency Medical Services (CECBEMS). AMLS course sites are not required to submit the CECBEMS continuing education fees because they are included in the AMLS surcharge fee. Further information on CECBEMS can be found at http://www.cecbems.org.

Provider and Instructor Recognition

Because medicine is ever changing, periodic revisions and updates will be required as the scientific and medical fields uncover new advances and techniques. Therefore, the AMLS provider, instructor, and affiliate faculty recognition is valid for four years.

Recognized Provider

The AMLS provider is one who has successfully completed the NAEMT AMLS Provider course and successfully passed both the cognitive and skills performance evaluation in accordance with the NAEMT and AMLS continuing educational course standards. Upon successful completion, the AMLS provider will be issued a certificate of completion that will be valid for four years. An AMLS Refresher course will renew AMLS provider recognition.

Use of Course Content

The Provider course complements the medical emergency module of the para-medic course Department of Transportation (DOT) curriculum. An AMLS course coordinator who chooses to use the AMLS Provider course materials within a paramedic program, or for continuing education classes in a modular form, may do so with the written permission of the NAEMT office and AMLS Executive Committee. The NAEMT course electronic application should reflect the actual beginning and ending course dates. The AMLS course scenarios and lecture presentations from the Provider course must be used as printed and not altered or edited.

Course Participants

Basic and advanced healthcare practioners may challenge the AMLS Provider and Refresher courses. Material covered will remain at the advanced level for all practioners. Advanced practioners, who qualify, may become eligible to become AMLS instructors.

Participant Prerequisites

Because AMLS is an advanced course that assumes a previous working knowl-edge of medical emergencies, there are necessary prerequisites. Course partici-pation is open to all providers: EMT-paramedics (EMT-Ps), EMT-intermediates (EMT-Is), EMT-basics (EMT-Bs), and to registered nurses (RNs) or physicians (MDs/DOs) and advanced level healthcare providers with at least one year of clinical experience. However, this is an advanced-level course and, as such, the participant must be academically and clinically prepared for a rapid-paced and thought-provoking class. This will ensure that participants have the base knowl-edge and experience on which the AMLS course will build. To successfully complete the course, the participant must read the AMLS textbook before the class and come to class prepared.

The course includes a separate pre-test and post-test written evaluation for EMT-basic providers. This allows more inclusion of basic level providers. Evaluation scenarios may be evaluated for competency at the basic level and will use the same evaluation tool as advanced providers. The need for advanced care should be appropriately recognized, and functioning as a team member during ALS care is essential.

Remediation and Re-Evaluation

Any participant who is unsuccessful in a component of the evaluation process in the Provider or Refresher course shall have the opportunity to be remediated and re-evaluated by the course coordinator or affiliate faculty. If remediation and re-evaluation is not conducted at the conclusion of the course, the participant shall have 30 days in which to complete the course competencies. Failure to comply with this timeframe will result in the participant's failure of the entire course.

NAEMT Surcharge

Upon completion of the Provider course, the course coordinator will submit to NAEMT the required surcharge of $15/participant for domestic and interna-tional courses and $10/participant for U.S. military courses.

Course Size

To maximize learning potential, class size is dependent on the instructor-patient-participant ratio. For each practical station, the highest ratio of instructor-patient to participant allowed will be one instructor to one patient for every five participants (1:1:5). Smaller ratios allow participants to have more time to practice and review each scenario. The success of the course relies on application of the didactic material to the physical assessment.

Instructor/Participant Ratio

The provider and instructor courses will use an instructor-patient-participant ratio of 1:1:5. This ratio will help ensure that all participants have ample opportunity to interact with the instructor and patient during practical scenarios. This process will enhance the participant's learning experience.

Post-Course Material

The course coordinator must ensure that all post-course paperwork and fees are submitted to NAEMT within 30 days of the completion of the course. Course coordinators who fail to comply will not be allowed to register for future courses until all outstanding paperwork and fees are received by the NAEMT office.

Electronic submission of pre-course and post-course materials for AMLS courses is required by NAEMT. The NAEMT education management software is provided by NAEMT free of charge. Course coordinators can access http://www.naemt.org/software or the NAEMT website to download the software.

The software is used to transmit the final roster of course participants. A summary of the course evaluations and instructor-monitoring forms will be mailed separately for each course. The appropriate NAEMT surcharge will also be mailed within 30 days of completion of the course. Provider, Refresher, and Instructor courses are considered separate courses, even if held on the same days.

Course Agenda

The course schedules have been developed to offer a proposed pattern for each course. The lecture content is specifically set to allow each instructor to build on concepts previously covered. This schedule should be closely adhered to. At no time should a lecture be moved or shortened without previous approval of the affiliate faculty and NAEMT. The proposed schedules are provided on the following pages. Schedule A includes the optional Airway Management scenario station.

A demonstration of the AMLS assessment process may be added to any of the AMLS courses schedules, where determined appropriate. Course coordinators should make a 10–15 minute adjustment in the following course schedules if they choose to add the demonstration component. Any AMLS instructor, course coordinator, or affiliate faculty member may participate in the demonstration.

SAMPLE SCHEDULE A

(Optional Airway Management Scenario Station)

Day 1

0730	Registration
0800	Introduction, Course Overview
0815	Lecture: Assessment of the Medical Patient
0915	Break
0930	Lecture: Airway Management, Ventilation, and Oxygen Therapy
1030	Group Rotations: Assessment (Scenario 1) and Airway (Scenario 1)
1130	Lecture: Hypoperfusion (Shock)
1230	Lunch
1315	Group Rotations: Hypoperfusion (Scenarios 1 to 4)
1435	Lecture: Dyspnea, Respiratory Distress, or Respiratory Failure
1535	Lecture: Chest Pain
1635	Group Rotations: Dyspnea (Scenarios 1 and 2) and Chest Pain (Scenarios 1 and 2)
1800	Adjourn

Day 2

0800	Lecture: Altered Mental Status
0900	Lecture: Abdominal Pain/GI Bleeding
1000	Break
1015	Group Rotations: Altered Mental Status (Scenarios 1 and 2) and Abdominal Pain/GI Bleeding (Scenarios 1 and 2)
1135	Pretest Review
1200	Lunch
1245	Final Exam Rotations—Four Evaluation Scenarios (Four topics: Dyspnea, Chest Pain, Altered Mental Status, and Abdominal Pain/GI Bleeding) and Written Exam
1545	Course Evaluation, Certificates/Cards Awarded

Group Rotations for 6–10 Participants

▶ Number of instructors: 4

▶ Group size: 3–5 participants per group

Day 1 *(with optional Airway Management Scenario)*

	1030–1100	1100–1130
Assessment (Scenario 1)	Group A	Group B
Airway (Scenario 1)	Group B	Group A
	1315–1355	**1355–1435**
Hypoperfusion (Scenarios 1 and 2)	Group A	Group B
Hypoperfusion (Scenarios 3 and 4)	Group B	Group A
	1635–1715	**1715–1755**
Dyspnea (Scenarios 1 and 2)	Group A	Group B
Chest Pain (Scenarios 1 and 2)	Group B	Group A

Day 2

	1015–1055	1055–1135
Altered Mental Status (Scenarios 1 and 2)	Group A	Group B
Abdominal Pain/GI Bleeding (Scenarios 1 and 2)	Group B	Group A

Final Exam Rotations for 6–10 Participants

▶ Number of instructors: 3–4

▶ Group size: 2–3 participants per group

▶ All evaluation stations are Scenario 4

Day 2

	1245–1315	1315–1345	1345–1415	1415–1445	1445–1515	1515–1545
Group A	Written	Written	I	II	III	IV
Group B	Written	Written	II	III	IV	I
Group C	I	II	III	IV	Written	Written

Key: I = Dyspnea; II = Chest Pain; III = Altered Mental Status; IV = Abdominal Pain/GI Bleeding

Group Rotations for 12–20 Participants

▶ Number of instructors: 4

▶ Group size: 3–5 participants per group

Day 1 (with optional Airway Management Scenarios)

	1030–1100	1100–1130		
Assessment (Scenario 1A)	Group A	Group C		
Assessment (Scenario 1B)	Group B	Group D		
Airway (Scenario 1A)	Group C	Group A		
Airway (Scenario 1B)	Group D	Group B		
	1315–1335	**1335–1355**	**1355–1415**	**1415–1435**
Hypoperfusion (Scenario 1)	Group A	Group B	Group C	Group D
Hypoperfusion (Scenario 2)	Group B	Group C	Group D	Group A
Hypoperfusion (Scenario 3)	Group C	Group D	Group A	Group B
Hypoperfusion (Scenario 4)	Group D	Group A	Group B	Group C
	1635–1715	**1715–1755**		
Dyspnea (Scenarios 1A and 2A)	Group A	Group C		
Dyspnea (Scenarios 1B and 2B)	Group B	Group D		
Chest Pain (Scenarios 1A and 2A)	Group C	Group A		
Chest Pain (Scenarios 1B and 2B)	Group D	Group B		

Day 2

	1015–1055	1055–1135
Altered Mental Status (Scenarios 1A and 2A)	Group A	Group C
Altered Mental Status (Scenarios 1B and 2B)	Group B	Group D
Abdominal Pain/GI Bleeding (Scenarios 1A and 2A)	Group C	Group A
Abdominal Pain/GI Bleeding (Scenarios 1B and 2B)	Group D	Group B

Final Exam Rotations for 12–20 Participants

▶ Number of instructors: 4–7

▶ Group size: 2–3 participants per group

▶ All evaluation stations are Scenario 4

Day 2

	1245–1315	1315–1345	1345–1415	1415–1445	1445–1515	1515–1545
Group A	Written	Written	I	II	III	IV
Group B	Written	Written	II	III	IV	I
Group C	I	II	III	IV	Written	Written
Group D	II	III	IV	I	Written	Written

Key: I = Dyspnea; II = Chest Pain; III = Altered Mental Status; IV = Abdominal Pain/GI Bleeding

SAMPLE SCHEDULE B

Day 1

0730	Registration
0800	Introduction, Course Overview
0810	Lecture: Assessment of the Medical Patient
0915	Break
0930	Lecture: Airway Management, Ventilation, and Oxygen Therapy Group Rotations: Assessment (Scenarios 1 and 2)
1030	Lecture: Hypoperfusion (Shock)
1130	Group Rotations: Hypoperfusion (Scenarios 1–4)
1230	Lunch
1315	Lecture: Chest Pain
1415	Break
1430	Lecture: Dyspnea, Respiratory Distress, Respiratory Failure
1530	Group Rotations: Dyspnea (Scenarios 1 and 2) and Chest Pain (Scenarios 1 and 2)
1630	Adjourn

Day 2

0800	Lecture: Altered Mental Status
0900	Break
0915	Lecture: Abdominal Pain/GI Bleeding
1015	Group Rotations: Altered Mental Status (Scenarios 1 and 2) and Abdominal Pain/GI Bleeding (Scenarios 1 and 2)
1115	Pretest Review
1200	Lunch
1245	Final Exam Rotations—Four Evaluation Scenarios (Four topics: Chest Pain, Dyspnea, Altered Mental Status, and Abdominal Pain/GI Bleeding) and Written Exam
1600	Course Evaluation, Certificates/Cards Awarded

Group Rotations for 6–10 Participants

▶ Number of instructors: 2

▶ Group size: 3–5 participants per group

Day 1

	1130–1200	1200–1230
Assessment (Scenarios 1 and 2)	Group A	Group B
Hypoperfusion (Scenarios 1 and 2)	Group B	Group A

	1530–1600	1600–1630
Dyspnea (Scenarios 1 and 2)	Group A	Group B
Chest Pain (Scenarios 1 and 2)	Group B	Group A

Day 2

	1015–1045	1045–1115
Altered Mental Status (Scenarios 1 and 2)	Group A	Group B
Abdominal Pain/GI Bleeding (Scenarios 1 and 2)	Group B	Group A

Final Exam Rotations for 6–10 Participants

▶ Number of instructors: 3–4

▶ Group size: 2–3 participants per group

▶ All evaluation stations are Scenario 4

Day 2

	1245–1315	1315–1345	1345–1415	1415–1445	1445–1515	1515–1545
Group A	Written	Written	I	II	III	IV
Group B	I	II	III	IV	Written	Written

Key: I = Chest Pain; II = Dyspnea; III = Altered Mental Status; IV = Abdominal Pain/GI Bleeding

Group Rotations for 12–20 Participants

▶ Number of instructors: 4

▶ Group size: 3–5 participants per group

NOTE: Scenario numbering 1A, 1B, etc. indicates same case scenario being presented simultaneously at two different stations.

Day 1

	1130–1200	1200–1230
Assessment (Scenarios 1A and 2A)	Group A	Group C
Assessment (Scenarios 1B and 2B)	Group B	Group D
Hypoperfusion (Scenarios 1A and 2A)	Group C	Group A
Hypoperfusion (Scenarios 1B and 2B)	Group D	Group B
	1530–1600	**1600–1630**
Dyspnea (Scenarios 1A and 2A)	Group A	Group C
Dyspnea (Scenarios 1B and 2B)	Group B	Group D
Chest Pain (Scenarios 1A and 2A)	Group C	Group A
Chest Pain (Scenarios 1B and 2B)	Group D	Group B

Day 2

	1015–1045	1045–1115
Altered Mental Status (Scenarios 1A and 2A)	Group A	Group C
Altered Mental Status (Scenarios 1B and 2B)	Group B	Group D
Abdominal Pain/GI Bleeding (Scenarios 1A and 2A)	Group C	Group A
Abdominal Pain/GI Bleeding (Scenarios 1B and 2B)	Group D	Group B

Final Exam Rotations for 12–20 Participants

▶ Number of instructors: 4–7

▶ Group size: 2–3 participants per group

▶ All evaluation stations are Scenario 4

	1245–1315	1315–1345	1345–1415	1415–1445	1445–1515	1515–1545
Group A	Written	Written	I	II	III	IV
Group B	Written	Written	II	III	IV	I
Group C	I	II	III	IV	Written	Written
Group D	II	III	IV	I	Written	Written

Key: I = Chest Pain; II = Dyspnea; III = Altered Mental Status; IV = Abdominal Pain/GI Bleeding

∷ INSTRUCTOR COURSE

Course Philosophy

The purpose of the Instructor course is to provide the AMLS instructor-candidate with the knowledge, skills, and support materials necessary to conduct and/or participate as faculty in an approved AMLS course. The course is designed to be an interactive lecture format that discusses the styles of adult learners, suggestions on maximizing the learning experience for participants, and the administration components of the AMLS courses.

The course is ideally conducted at the conclusion of an AMLS Provider course; however, it can be taught as a stand-alone course. It is essential to disseminate the course philosophy and content consistent with the standards established by NAEMT and the AMLS Executive Committee. No deviations in content are allowed. Any removal or addition of slides, equipment, materials, or structure of the Instructor course requires approval in advance and in writing to the AMLS chairperson. Approval should not be assumed. Approval, if granted, will be submitted in writing to the requesting individual.

The AMLS Instructor course is designed to be a 4-hour course for those who have achieved instructor-candidate potential when successfully completing an AMLS Provider or Refresher course. Course participants who are advanced practioners may obtain instructor-candidate potential by:

- ▶ Completion of the post-test with a minimum score of 84%
- ▶ Obtaining a superior rating in the four evaluation stations
- ▶ Holding an advanced healthcare provider status
- ▶ Having experience teaching at an advanced practioner level

An Instructor course can be held following a Provider course or as a stand-alone course. After completion of the course, the participant is considered an AMLS instructor if the following criteria are met:

- ▶ Successful completion of the AMLS Instructor course
- ▶ Successfully monitored by AMLS affiliate faculty within one year of attendance of an AMLS instructor course

Course Application

The AMLS Instructor course application is completed on-line using the NAEMT educational management software or NAEMT website a minimum of 60 days prior to the course date.

Continuing Education Credits

The continuing education credits are nationally approved by the NAEMT organizational accreditation by the Continuing Education Coordinating Board of Emergency Medical Services (CECBEMS). Four (4) hours of continuing education are awarded for the Instructor course.

Instructor Course Faculty

Each course will be conducted by an AMLS affiliate faculty member.

Upon completion of the Instructor course, the affiliate faculty will issue the Instructor certificate and wallet card. Therefore, the certificate and wallet card are issued on the same day as completion of the course.

Instructor Recognition

In order to obtain instructor status, an instructor-candidate must be monitored lecturing and teaching in the skill stations in a Provider or Refresher course. Affiliate faculty will submit the monitoring forms to NAEMT. The affiliate faculty member may also give the candidate's successful monitoring form to the course coordinator to submit with any post-course paperwork.

The instructor recognition is valid for four years. AMLS instructors are required to teach a minimum of one course per year to maintain their instructor status.

Successful completion of the Instructor course process enables new instructors to teach Provider and Refresher courses using the AMLS philosophy and guidelines. Individuals selected to attend this course are typically experienced instructors and must have current status as a healthcare provider with clinical skills and knowledge at an advanced level.

Course Materials

Each instructor-candidate participant must receive a current edition of the *AMLS Coordinator & Instructor Guide.* The Guide will be reviewed during the course administration component of the course.

NAEMT Surcharge

The NAEMT surcharge for the Instructor course is $10/participant for domestic, international, and U.S. military courses.

Instructor/Participant Ratio

No minimum instructor-to-participant ratio is required for the Instructor course.

Post-Course Paperwork

Post-course paperwork submission is the same as for a Provider or Refresher course.

Course Agenda

0845   Registration

0900   Welcome/Introduction

       AMLS Textbook and Coordinator Instructor Guide Recognition

       Goals and Objectives of the AMLS Instructor Course

1000   Break

1010   Course Philosophy

       Moving the Practioner from an Assessment-Based Model to a Diagnostic-Based Model

       Mentoring Critical Thinking Skills/Teaching Adult Learners

1100   Break

1110   Use of the *AMLS Coordinator & Instructor Guide*

Enhancing scenarios in group practical settings

Role of the AMLS faculty

Interactive lecture presentations

Course coordination

▣ REFRESHER COURSE

Course Philosophy

The course incorporates scenario-based, interactive lectures and evaluation stations. It is essential to disseminate the course philosophy and content consistent with the standards established by NAEMT and the AMLS Executive Committee. No deviations in content are acceptable. Any removal or addition of slides, equipment, materials, or structure of the Refresher course requires approval in advance and in writing to the AMLS chairperson. Approval should not be assumed. Approval, if granted, will be submitted in writing to the requesting course coordinator.

Prerequisites for Participants

The AMLS Refresher course is designed to be a 4-hour course. It is offered to current AMLS providers who are nearing the expiration of their 4-year recognition. A Refresher course must be taken prior to the provider recognition expiration date.

If an individual is unable to take a Refresher course, course coordinators and/or affiliate faculty can admit an individual into a scheduled Refresher course up to six months past their expiration date if the AMLS provider's medical director requires they maintain AMLS provider recognition, have been deployed to serve in the military, or injury or illness has prevented their attendance. This will not change their expiration date; it will only reflect the extended period within which an individual will be allowed into a Refresher course. Participants who seek to reinstate their term of recognition after their expiration date are required to attend a full Provider course. Individuals may not attend the second day of a Provider course to fulfill the Refresher course requirement.

Continuing Education Credits

The continuing education credits are nationally approved by the NAEMT organizational accreditation by the Continuing Education Coordinating Board of Emergency Medical Services (CECBEMS). Four hours of continuing education are awarded for the Refresher course.

Successful Completion

Successful completion requires:

▶ Attendance for the entire course

▶ Competency in the four evaluation stations: Altered Mental Status, Chest Pain (includes Hypoperfusion), Dyspnea/Respiratory Failure, and Abdominal Pain/GI Bleeding.

▶ A minimum score of 76% on the written evaluation

An AMLS certificate and wallet card will be awarded by the course coordinator and/or affiliate faculty upon successful completion. Provider status recognition is for four years.

Course Application

The AMLS Refresher course application is completed on-line using the NAEMT educational management software or NAEMT website a minimum of 60 days prior to the course date.

The Refresher course may be co-located within the second day of a Provider course or done as a stand-alone course and requires a separate course application. If co-located within the second day of a Provider course, the lecture portion will be done simultaneously during the morning portion. Both groups of participants will be brought together for the evaluation components.

Required Participant Materials

Participants must have a copy of the current edition of the *Advanced Medical Life Support* textbook and copies of the appropriate pre-course materials. Pre-course materials should be sent to each participant a minimum of 30 days prior to the course. The AMLS pre-test must be completed prior to the beginning of the course.

Remediation

Any participant unsuccessful in the evaluation components of the Refresher course will be awarded the same opportunity for remediation and re-evaluation as indicated in a Provider course.

NAEMT Surcharge

The NAEMT surcharge for the Refresher course is $10/participant for domestic, international, and U.S. military courses.

Instructor/Participant Ratio

The provider and instructor courses will use an instructor-patient-participant ratio of 1:1:5. This ratio will assist in assuring all participants have ample opportunity to interact with the instructor and patient during practical scenarios. This process will enhance the participant's learning experience.

Post-Course Paperwork

Post-course paperwork submission is the same as a Provider or Instructor course.

Course Agenda

(Incorporated with second day of Provider course using Schedule A):

0830   Registration

0900   Welcome/Introduction

0915	AMLS Refresher Review Presentation—Part I
1020	Break
1035	AMLS Refresher Review Presentation—Part II
1135	Review of Pretest
1200	Lunch
1245	Group Evaluation Rotations in Dyspnea, Chest Pain, Altered Mental Status, and Abdominal Pain/GI Bleeding. (Scenario 4 will be used for all evaluation stations. Chest Pain Scenario 4 encompasses hypoperfusion. Scenario 3 can be used for retesting situations after remediation.)

The written exam is also taken at an evaluation station.

1545	Course Evaluation/Cards Awarded

(Incorporated with second day of Provider Course using Schedule B):

0815	Registration
0845	Welcome/Introduction
0900	AMLS Refresher Review Presentation—Part I
1000	Break
1015	AMLS Refresher Review Presentation—Part II
1115	Review of Pretest
1200	Lunch
1245	Group Evaluation Rotations in Dyspnea, Chest Pain, Altered Mental Status, and Abdominal Pain/GI Bleeding. (Scenario 4 will be used for all evaluation stations. Chest Pain Scenario 4 encompasses hypoperfusion. Scenario 3 can be used for retesting situations after remediation.)

The written exam is also an evaluation station.

1545	Course Evaluation/Cards Awarded

Stand-Alone Course

0730	Registration
0800	Welcome/Introduction
0810	AMLS Refresher Review Presentation—Part I
0900	Break
0910	AMLS Refresher Review Presentation—Part II
1010	Break
1020	Review of Pretest
1030	Group Evaluation Rotations in Dyspnea, Chest Pain, Altered Mental Status, and Abdominal Pain/GI Bleed. (Scenario 4 will be used for all evaluation stations. Chest Pain Scenario 4 encompasses hypoperfusion. Scenario 3 can be used for retesting situations after remediation.)
1130	Written Exam

Instructor Update

The AMLS textbook, this *Coordinator & Instructor Guide,* and the accompanying NAEMT course CD-ROM will be reviewed and revised on a continuous basis. New information will be published as new science and trends unfold in our ever-changing medical field. Information regarding these changes will be forwarded to instructors and affiliate faculty by memorandum, or electronically or by required attendance at an AMLS Instructor Update workshop. The process will be determined as the need arises and at the guidance of NAEMT and the AMLS Executive Committee. If deemed necessary, there will be a phase-in period during which the previous edition will still be available for those who have not attended an update workshop or for course sites whose course schedules require extended timeframes.

AMLS instructors, course coordinators, affiliate/state, military, and international faculty will be advised on an onging basis of new policies and procedures and course materials electronically, via memorandums, the NAEMT website, and NAEMT News publications.

Course Materials

AMLS Text and Instructor Resources   The required textbook for this course is *Advanced Medical Life Support,* 3rd Ed., published by Brady/Prentice Hall. This textbook will serve as the primary resource throughout the course. Each participant must receive a copy of the textbook at least one month in advance of the course. The textbook gives the participant the fundamental background and is essential for successful course completion.

In order to ensure consistency in the delivery of material, no deviation from the prescribed NAEMT/AMLS course content or policies will be allowed. The course coordinator must ensure that the textbook is obtained. The AMLS textbook can be ordered directly from Brady/Prentice Hall or at http://www.EMSBooks.com.

This *AMLS Coordinator & Instructor Guide* is an invaluable resource for the instructor who teaches the Provider, Instructor, or Refresher AMLS courses. This publication provides the necessary instructor resources to obtain the instructor notes for lecture presentations, scenarios for the hands-on practical, and guidance for the administrative components of the courses. Forms used in the course that do not appear within the NAEMT course software are also included. This Guide includes a summary of the course objectives for each topic covered in the various scenarios. The scenarios in this Guide are intended to be used with the appropriate assessment stations. AMLS instructors teaching the practical stations will use the scenarios in this guide. These scenarios can be duplicated from the text for distribution to the AMLS instructors to assist them as they mentor the individuals used as patients in the various practical stations. The beginning of each scenario includes a list of required equipment for that station as well as referenced chapters from the associated AMLS textbook. It is imperative to use the required equipment and live patients. This practice offers the participants the opportunity to actively apply the assessment techniques and provides real-time communication and patient management throughout the scenarios.

Pre-course materials, such as handouts and pre- and post-tests, are obtained from the NAEMT office by the on-site coordinator when a course application is approved and issued a national course number. The course coordinator will send the handouts to the participants, along with the AMLS textbook, a minimum of 30 days prior to the course date. Duplication of all materials will be the responsibility of the hosting organization. The security of the post-tests must be ensured to prevent any possibility of compromising the integrity of the tests.

The AMLS PowerPoint® slide presentations for the Provider, Instructor, and Refresher courses are provided by NAEMT. This CD-ROM is obtained from NAEMT when a course application is approved. Only AMLS-recognized course coordinators and affiliate faculty are eligible to receive the CD-ROM. At this time, there is no fee for the CD-ROM. The CD-ROM may not be duplicated in its entirety for course instructors or used within other programs. Instructors with lecture assignments will receive their lecture presentation only for course preparation. The NAEMT CD-ROM is used solely for the lecture presentations of the AMLS Provider, Instructor, and Refresher courses.

Educators may purchase additional AMLS audio-visual materials for use in other courses through Brady Publishing. These materials can be used in conjunction with the AMLS textbook, but are not used with the established AMLS courses.

The Provider and Refresher courses are intended to be a real-time, interactive experience for the participant. Participants will communicate with real patients and/or bystanders for each practical scenario. Treatment interventions should also be done in a real-time format. For example, blood pressure cuffs, IV therapy, and cardiac monitors should be used with the appropriate equipment in each station. The instructor will moderate the discussion points that are identified in each scenario. Minimal moulage and simulated vomit should be used in all Provider and Refresher courses. Equipment requirements for practical station are listed at the beginning of each scenario.

▦ COURSE REQUIREMENTS

Live Patients

A minimum of four live patients are required for all provider and refresher courses. A combination of both male and female patients is ideal. Course coordinators are responsible for ensuring the patients are well informed about the scenarios they will be participating in. Manikins may be used for scenarios where an unconscious patient is designated.

Equipment Requirements

Although AMLS is a highly interactive course, the practical scenarios require minimal equipment. There are four practical stations for a course of 20–26 participants. All scenario stations need to have the following equipment:

- ▶ Tracheal intubation, and LMA®, PtL®, and Combitube® airway equipment
- ▶ Nasal cannula, non-rebreather mask, bag-valve-mask (BVM), oral/nasal airways, nebulizer kit, and color metric end-tidal CO_2 detector
- ▶ Blood pressure cuff, stethoscope, pulse oximeter, blood glucose monitor, pen light, emesis basin, and blanket
- ▶ Cardiac monitor and simulator

▶ Minimal moulage and a live patient

▶ IV therapy adjuncts (normal saline, dopamine, IV tubing, tape)

▶ Table/chairs for instructor and patient

▶ Chairs for participants

▶ Sample medications relevant to the differential diagnoses

AMLS Course Evaluation Tools

The AMLS Executive Committee is responsible for the development and quality of the written evaluation tools. There is a pre- and post-test for each basic and advanced level practioner. The basic and advanced level written evaluations have the same content areas. However, the questions and distracters are written to either a basic or advanced scope of practice. Course coordinators must request copies of the basic written evaluations at the time of course application. Advanced level written evaluations will automatically be sent with each approved course.

The most current written evaluations must be used in the Provider and Refresher courses. This evaluation tool is revised on an ongoing basis. Course coordinators and affiliate faculty will be notified of revisions. The revised versions will be sent to course coordinators as courses are scheduled and approved. Minimum competency on the written evaluation is 76% for all provider levels.

Course sites may be asked to participate in a written evaluation of the tool validation process. This process will be ongoing with each revision of the tools.

Discrepancies in the written evaluation may be forwarded to the NAEMT international office.

Final evaluation scenarios must not be altered in any way. The AMLS course uses Scenario #4 for each of the practical evaluation stations. The four evaluation stations are: Dyspnea/Respiratory Failure, Chest Pain (includes Hypoperfusion), Altered Mental Status, and Abdominal Pain/GI Bleeding.

If a participant does not meet the minimum competency in an evaluation station, the content should be remediated. The participant is awarded the opportunity for re-evaluation. The participant will be re-evaluated on similar topic area, but with Scenario #3.

Education Management Software

Use of the NAEMT education management software is required for all AMLS courses. This software is provided by NAEMT, free of charge. All course applications, pre-course, and post-course required records must be transmitted via the software to NAEMT. The software can be found at http://www.naemt.org/software.

Course Budget

It is the responsibility of the course coordinator to collect course fees, identify the hosting facility, equipment, and refreshments. The course coordinator will arrange payment for any instructor costs. The coordinator will obtain all required course equipment.

The NAEMT surcharge is $15 per person for the Provider course, $10 per participant for the Instructor course, and $10 per participant for the Refresher course. All U.S. military courses will be charged an additional $10/participant.

When determining course cost, figure in the cost of the following:

- ▶ NAEMT surcharge
- ▶ Facility fee
- ▶ Instructor honoraria
- ▶ Patient honoraria
- ▶ Additional course faculty honoraria
- ▶ Textbooks
- ▶ Audiovisual expenses
- ▶ Printing cost—pre- and post-tests, course handouts, etc.
- ▶ Advertisements
- ▶ Postage for mailings
- ▶ Refreshments
- ▶ Additional materials

The cost for an inaugural course may be higher due to travel expenses for your faculty or the import of instructors/affiliate faculty to your location. Identifying local faculty and equipment for future courses will reduce course costs. Many of the above costs may also be eliminated if the hosting organization can provide the facility, instructors, audiovisual equipment, and copying for the AMLS courses.

Course Paperwork

The course coordinators are responsible for the timely submission of post-course paperwork and fees to NAEMT. NAEMT requires payment of all surcharge fees and paperwork within 30 days of completion of the course. Course coordinators, affiliate faculty or course sites who are deficient in submitting payment or paperwork within the designated time frame may be denied further course approval for delinquent items. This decision is at the discretion of NAEMT. An individual course coordinator, affiliate faculty, or state or international coordinator status may be removed if consistent violation of NAEMT and AMLS course policies and procedures occurs.

Course Application

A proposed course application will need to be approved by NAEMT 60 days in advance. Within 30 days of the course, a confirmation letter with course materials will be sent to the course coordinator. This letter will confirm that the course has been approved and registered. All registered courses will be placed on the AMLS website. The proposed course application should include the:

- ▶ Name of the hosting organization
- ▶ Names of the course coordinator, affiliate faculty, instructors, and medical director
- ▶ Location and time frame of the course

- Agenda with AMLS instructor assignments
- Anticipated number of participants

NAEMT will review the proposed application for approval and registration. Upon approval, a national course number will be issued and the appropriate pre-course materials forwarded to the course coordinator. Pre-course materials include, but are not limited to:

- Pre-test
- Pre-test annotated answer sheet
- Post-test I
- Participant answer sheet
- Post-test I annotated answer sheet
- Assessment handout
- Math calculation handout

Participant Application

The participant registration form must be filled out by each participant. The participant registration form information must be entered into the NAEMT software upon completion of the course. The form must include all pertinent and required sections to be completed. This includes the participant's name, address, telephone number, written evaluation score, and whether the participant passed or failed the evaluation stations. The participant's information is transmitted electronically via the NAEMT software. The NAEMT surcharge must be sent via mail, directly to the NAEMT office.

Course Certificates and Cards

Upon completion of the course, the course coordinator must send the appropriate course paperwork within 30 days to NAEMT. The AMLS certificates and wallet cards are sent from the NAEMT international office to the course coordinator/affiliate faculty when a course is registered. Participants should be awarded the appropriate certificate and card upon successful completion of the course. The course coordinator or affiliate faculty has the responsibility of distributing them to all appropriate course participants at the completion of the course. At no time should certificates and cards be mailed at a date after the conclusion of the course.

Course Evaluations

Each participant will be required to fill out a course evaluation. Course evaluations should be submitted for Provider, Instructor, and Refresher courses. You may use a summary format to submit the scores and comments to NAEMT along with other post-course paperwork. They may also be sent electronically. These forms can be found in Section III in this manual.

Instructor Evaluations

Instructor evaluations may be completed by participants as deemed appropriate by the course coordinator, affiliate faculty, and medical director. Each instructor should be given the opportunity to review these evaluations. These evaluations do not need to be forwarded to NAEMT with the post-course paperwork unless the course coordinator, affiliate faculty, or medical director deem appropriate. These forms can be found in Section III in this manual.

Maintenance of Records

All course materials must be kept on file for a minimum of five years. This will ensure compliance with CECBEMS continuing education credit records requirement.

⊞ COURSE FACULTY

Faculty Requirements

All course faculty must be AMLS-recognized instructors. Each program must have the following faculty:

▶ One on-site course coordinator

▶ One on- or off-site medical director

    ▶ The medical director must be available by phone during all courses

▶ One on- or off-site affiliate faculty

    ▶ Affiliate faculty must be present if instructor-candidates are to be monitored. They may be available by phone during all other courses.

Faculty-to-Participant Ratios

AMLS Provider and Refresher courses require a high level of participation and interaction by the instructors and participants. Lecture and practical scenarios require significant hands-on, real-time simulated patient/student interaction. Therefore, it is imperative that practical scenarios have one instructor and one patient for every five students (1:1:5).

AMLS Instructor

The AMLS instructor is the core, or backbone, of the educational component of this course. AMLS instructors who serve as faculty must have completed the AMLS instructor-candidate course and been monitored by AMLS affiliate faculty within a year of that course. The AMLS instructor recognition is valid for four years and requires that the instructor teach a minimum of one course each year. Instructors need to be competent in the lecture presentations and skill stations. AMLS instructors should be used in their area of expertise. Instructors are accountable to the AMLS executive committee, course coordinators, and affiliate faculty.

Qualifications The AMLS instructor must:

▶ Have completed an AMLS Provider or Refresher course and received an instructor potential rating. (An instructor potential rating is acquired by achieving an 84% or higher on the Provider course written exam and a superior rating on one's performance in the teaching and evaluation stations.) Completion of the instructor course recognizes an individual as an instructor-candidate.

▶ Have previous instructional experience in teaching PHTLS, advanced cardiac life support (ACLS), pediatric advanced life support (PALS), or equivalent advanced level courses.

▶ Have current status as an advanced healthcare professional/provider.

▶ Teach in at least one AMLS course per year during their four-year recognition term.

Responsibilities   The AMLS instructor is required to:

▶ Be monitored by an affiliate faculty member within one year of becoming an instructor-candidate.

▶ Affiliate faculty will provide the course coordinator with the Instructor-Candidate Monitoring form which will be submitted with the Provider or Refresher post-course paperwork. NAEMT will then register the individual as an instructor.

▶ Adhere to all NAEMT/AMLS policies and procedures to ensure course security and integrity.

▶ Maintain competence in knowledge and skills in all assignments for AMLS courses.

▶ Participate in teaching lecture presentations and skill stations.

▶ Complete the necessary documentation for the practical stations.

▶ Report any necessary information regarding course participant's performance to the course coordinator or affiliate faculty member.

▶ Remain an instructor in good standing.

▶ Assist the course coordinators in course management with tasks involving: equipment set-up and take-down, moulage of patients, ensuring that patients understand assigned station scenarios, evaluation of participant performance, and completion of participant evaluation forms.

▶ Inform the course coordinator, affiliate faculty, or medical director of any conflict that arises during the course.

Course Coordinator

The course coordinator is responsible for overseeing the day-to-day operations of each individual course. This person is ultimately the key to the success of this course. Course coordinators serve at the appointment of the AMLS Executive Committee and/or state coordinator. The course coordinator is responsible for answering any questions that may arise, resolving conflict, ensuring that proper station equipment is available and that live patients participate in all teaching and evaluation stations, and handling administrative duties for the course. In rare instances, the course coordinator may not be recognized as an AMLS instructor or affiliate faculty. Permission from NAEMT and the AMLS Executive Committee will be required in this instance. Course coordinators are accountable to the AMLS Executive Committee, affiliate faculty, and/or state coordinator.

Qualifications   The course coordinator must have:

▶ Successfully completed the AMLS Provider and Instructor courses.

▶ Previous administrative experience coordinating PHTLS, basic trauma life support (BTLS), ACLS, PALS, pediatric education for prehospital professionals (PEPP), or similar courses at the advanced level.

▶ Access to the necessary equipment, live patients, and facilities that are vital to providing a quality program.

Responsibilities   The course coordinator is required to:

▶ Electronically submit via the NAEMT management software or NAEMT website course applications and post-course transmissions.

▶ Distribute all pre-course packets for participants and determine AMLS faculty to teach in the course and monitor instructor-candidates.

▶ Ensure that all post-course paperwork is submitted to NAEMT within 30 days of course completion. Failure to comply will inhibit course activity until outstanding issues are resolved per NAEMT and AMLS policy and procedure. The post-course paperwork includes:

— Instructor monitoring forms

— Summary of course evaluations

— Participant data transmission

— NAEMT surcharge

▶ Plan, budget, and organize course equipment, faculty, patients, and participants in an efficient and timely manner.

▶ Collect and submit the NAEMT surcharge per participant. Checks are payable to NAEMT. (There is a surcharge of $15/Provider course participant, $10/Instructor course participant, $10/Refresher course participant, and $10/participant for all U.S. military courses.)

▶ Submit post-course material via the NAEMT software or website within 30 days of the course completion. Each course type must be registered separately. Post-course information will be transmitted separately. The information on the participant registration form must be transmitted.

▶ Adhere to all NAEMT/AMLS policies and procedures and standards to ensure course security and integrity.

▶ Identify on the course application the on-site hosting organization.

▶ Coordinate and/or teach a minimum of one course per year.

▶ Submit a summary of the course evaluations to the NAEMT international office and appropriate affiliate faculty and/or state coordinators.

AMLS Affiliate Faculty

The AMLS affiliate faculty are responsible for overseeing all the AMLS programs in their geographic area, state, or country/province. The affiliate faculty are also responsible for making decisions, along with NAEMT, concerning possible changes in course material to meet local protocols; ensuring that course coordinators are performing their jobs; and acting as a direct extension of

NAEMT for the AMLS course. Affiliate faculty are appointed by the AMLS Executive Committee and/or state coordinator. Affifliate faculty are accountable to the AMLS Executive Committee, course coordinator, and state coordinators.

Qualifications needed for appointment to affiliate faculty recognition include:

▶ Proof of recognition as a monitored AMLS instructor in good standing.

▶ The time and ability to devote to monitoring and/or supervising area courses.

▶ Proof of current and maintained NAEMT membership status.

▶ Letter of recommendation from local medical director, AMLS affiliate faculty, or state coordinator.

▶ Experience teaching and coordinating a minimum of one Provider course with a satisfactory evaluation from AMLS affiliate faculty.

▶ Recommendations for affiliate faculty status are submitted to the NAEMT office. Upon approval, the AMLS chairperson and/or state coordinator will appoint the individual to receive AMLS affiliate faculty recognition. Individuals will receive notification by letter from the AMLS chairperson and/or State coordinator.

Responsibilities   The affiliate faculty are required to:

▶ Assist with curriculum development and implementation.

▶ Be available or on-site during the course. Medical direction should also be accessible during the course.

▶ Teach and participate in a minimum of one course each year.

▶ Provide remediation in lieu of the course coordinator or medical director.

▶ Monitor instructor-candidates and ensure their Instructor Monitor form is submitted with the post-course paperwork.

▶ Adhere to all NAEMT/AMLS standards to ensure course quality and integrity.

▶ Communicate with the state coordinator all course activity and course summary evaluations. Identify and collaborate on any conflict issues.

▶ Teach and coordinate required instructor workshop updates for recognized AMLS course coordinators and instructors as directed by the AMLS Executive Committee and/or state coordinator.

Course Medical Director

A medical director is a very important aspect of this course. The medical director will give guidance to participants and faculty on issues that are brought to their attention regarding AMLS philosophy, course content, and rationale regarding current science and patient care issues. The medical director should have some involvement in training, educating, or directing EMS providers and basic and advanced healthcare practitioners in his or her geographic area. This will allow the physician to be familiar with the current local standards/operational orders in prehospital emergency care. Each medical director must be approved by the region's affiliate faculty and/or state coordinator to ensure that the necessary requirements are met. The course medical director may be offsite, but must be available during the course to answer questions and provide medical direction. Course medical directors are accountable to the AMLS Executive Committee and course and state/provincial coordinators.

Qualifications   The medical director must be:

▶ A licensed practicing physician (MD or DO)

▶ Actively involved in prehospital emergency medicine or currently practice in a primary care area of medicine and have an interest in EMS

Responsibilities   The medical director is required to:

▶ Ensure the accuracy of all medical-related course information.

▶ Serve as a resource personnel, answering questions for faculty and participants.

▶ Act together with the affiliate faculty and/or state coordinator, course coordinator, and instructors to resolve any problems or conflicts during the course. Assist with a participants or instructor remediation where designated by course coordinators, affiliate faculty, and/or state coordinators.

▶ Adhere to the NAEMT/AMLS course policies/procedures, guidelines, and standards.

▶ Participate as faculty for lecture presentations, when possible.

Adjunct Course Faculty

Additional course faculty are course members who are not necessarily AMLS instructors or providers, but act as integral members of the AMLS team. These team members may include medical directors or licensed physicians. The adjunct faculty is accountable to the course coordinator.

Qualifications   Adjunct Course Faculty

The adjunct faculty:

▶ Are selected by the course coordinator

▶ Must be a licensed, practicing physician with emergency and prehospital experience

▶ Must have knowledge in the AMLS philosophy, assessment, and management of patients with medical emergencies

Responsibilities   The adjunct course faculty is responsible for:

▶ Adhering to the NAEMT/AMLS policies/procedures, standards, and guidelines for all programs

▶ Assisting with the lecture presentations

State/International Coordinators

State or international coordinators are appointed by the AMLS chairperson, in collaboration with the AMLS Executive Committee. These coordinators are responsible for the maintenance of the integrity and quality of the AMLS courses. State or international coordinators are accountable to the NAEMT and AMLS chairperson.

Qualifications   The state or international coordinator must:

▶ Maintain current membership with NAEMT

▶ Provide documentation of current AMLS instructor and/or affiliate faculty status

▶ Commit to the administrative and/or course coordinator function as state or international coordinator

▶ Have experience in oversight of medical professionals, both prehospital and in-hospital

▶ Sign an NAEMT conflict of interest statement and be free of any conflicting interests, financial or otherwise, that would inhibit the promotion or mission of AMLS

▶ Submit a professional CV indicating work and educational experience to the AMLS chairperson

Responsibilities   The state and international coordinators will be responsible for:

▶ Recognizing and actively recruiting sites to host AMLS courses.

▶ Informing recognized AMLS instructors, affiliate faculty, and course coordinators of policies, procedures, and change in guidelines for all AMLS courses.

▶ Maintaining professional relationships with diverse healthcare and educational institutions in their state/province/country.

▶ Evaluating and recommending AMLS instructors for affiliate faculty and course coordinator status.

▶ Collaborating with AMLS sites within their state/province/country for reports as requested by NAEMT or the AMLS Executive Committee

▶ Providing conflict resolution with AMLS issues within their state/province/country.

▶ Maintaining quality assurance in all AMLS programs held in their state/province/country.

▶ Serving as national faculty for instructor/coordinator updates and workshops at the direction of NAEMT and/or the AMLS chairperson.

▶ Advising the AMLS international office and AMLS chairperson of new appointments to affiliate faculty status.

▶ Promoting course activity and quality assurance only within their own state/province/country.

▶ Evaluating current course materials and contributing to the development of a more acceptable statewide, provincial, or international AMLS course product. Input on recommendations for future revisions of course material to accomplish this goal will be forwarded in writing to the AMLS chairperson.

U.S. Military Coordinator

The AMLS chairperson will appoint military coordinators who coordinate all components of courses in the U.S. Military. This recognition is valid for four years. Military coordinators are accountable to the NAEMT and AMLS chairperson.

Qualifications   Military Coordinator

The military course coordinator qualifications require:

▶ Current and maintained membership with NAEMT

▶ Current AMLS instructor or affiliate faculty status

▶ Commitment to serve the administrative responsibilities of AMLS programs

▶ Letter of recommendation from their superior commanding officer

▶ Signing an NAEMT conflict of interest form and be free from any potential conflicts of interest

Responsibilities   The military coordinator will be responsible for:

▶ Communication with the AMLS chairperson.

▶ Recommending instructor-candidates for affiliate faculty and course coordinator status.

▶ Implementing new policies and procedures and content updates with military AMLS instructors and affiliate faculty.

▶ Submitting NAEMT or AMLS chairperson delegated reports in a timely manner to the AMLS international office.

▶ Promoting AMLS courses within the diverse military disciplines.

▶ Serving as national faculty for instructor and affiliate faculty updates and workshops at the discretion of NAEMT policy and the AMLS chairperson.

▶ Evaluating current course materials and contributing to the development of a more acceptable military personnel compatable AMLS course product. Input on recommendations for future revisions of course material to accomplish this goal will be forwarded in writing to the AMLS chairperson.

Patients

All Provider and Refresher courses need a minimum of four individuals who will serve as patients for the teaching and evaluation stations. This will enhance the learning process by allowing participants some real-time hands-on practice with the assessment skills. There should be a mixture of both male and female patients to compliment the scenarios.

Qualifications   The patient must meet the following qualifications:

▶ It is preferred if patients have a background in healthcare. Training at a minimum of an EMT-basic student is preferred.

▶ The ability and willingness to role play assigned scenarios.

Responsibilities   The patient is required to:

▶ Accurately portray a patient with a specific set of pathophysiologic conditions

▶ Interact with participants and the assessment evaluator as needed

▶ Accept minimal moulage relavent to scenario station assignment

Hosting Organization

The local hosting organization has many different roles and responsibilities that need to be fulfilled in order for the course to be a success.

Responsibilities   The hosting organization must:

▶ Provide adequate facilities for the course, which include, but are not limited to, a lecture room with adequate seating for all participants, rooms in which to conduct practical examinations, restroom facilities, and appropriate equipment for each practical scenario.

▶ Provide AMLS instructors, patients, and a medical director for the course.

▶ Work closely with local AMLS and EMS representatives to advertise the course appropriately.

▶ Develop a working budget to allow for necessary expenses, such as the cost of travel and honorariums for faculty.

▶ Assume the administrative responsibilities necessary for the granting of state-required continuing education hours. CECBEMS awards sixteen hours of continuing medical education (CME) for the AMLS Provider Course, and four hours for each Instructor and Refresher course. The CECBEMS National CME number is assigned with each approved course application.

▶ Assume the revenue responsibilities, including student registration, course confirmation, texts, student manuals and handouts, and submission of the NAEMT surcharge appropriate per participant for the designated course.

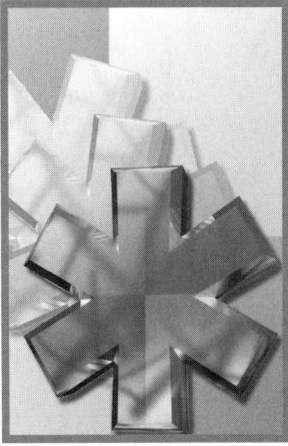

III. ADVANCED MEDICAL LIFE SUPPORT COURSE FORMS

▦ MEDICAL LIFE SUPPORT COURSE FORMS

The following forms are provided:

- ▶ Advanced Medical Life Support Course Budget
- ▶ Advanced Medical Life Support Course Evaluation Form
- ▶ Advanced Medical Life Support Instructor Evaluation Form
- ▶ Advanced Medical Life Support Instructor-Candidate Monitoring Form
- ▶ Advanced Medical Life Support Participant Final Evaluation Form
- ▶ Advanced Medical Life Support Participant Exam Answer Sheet
- ▶ Advanced Medical Life Support Provider Course Evaluation Summary Sheet
- ▶ Advanced Medical Life Support Course Roster
- ▶ NAEMT Advanced Medical Life Support Participant Registration Form
- ▶ Advanced Medical Life Support Instructor Roster

Advanced Medical Life Support
Course Budget

Course date(s): _____ Sponsor: _____

Submitted by: _____ Date: _____

EXPENSES

Personnel

Lecturers		
Skill station instructors		
Patients/moulage		
Secretarial support		
Other:		

Affiliate Faculty (as applicable)

Travel		
Lodging		
Meals		

Facilities

Facility charge		
Meals		
Refreshments		
Other:		

Materials, Equipment, and Supplies

Equipment rental		
Supplies		
Printing/duplication		
Brochures		
Postage		
Textbooks		
Other:		

NAEMT Surcharge

Provider: $15 × _____		
Instructor: $10 × _____		
Refresher: $10 × _____		
Military: $10 × _____		

REVENUES

Tuition fee $ _____ × _____ participants		
Textbooks sold		
Meals fee (if charged)		
Other:		

TOTAL EXPENSES   _____

TOTAL REVENUES   _____

NET   _____

ADVANCED MEDICAL LIFE SUPPORT
COURSE EVALUATION FORM

National Course #: _____ Course Location: _____

Country of Course Location: _____ ☐ Domestic ☐ Military

Course Date(s): _____ Course Type: ☐ Provider ☐ Refresher ☐ Instructor

Healthcare Provider Level (Circle One)

Physician   Physician Assistant   Adv. Nurse Practitioner   Registered Nurse   EMT-Basic
    Paramedic   Other: _____

Please rate the following aspects of the course. The following scale will be utilized:

1—Excellent
2—Good
3—Fair
4—Adequate

1) Overall evaluation of the course	1 2 3 4
2) Overall presentation of lecture material	1 2 3 4
3) Overall knowledge of course faculty	1 2 3 4
4) Overall rating of the facility	1 2 3 4
5) Overall rating of the audiovisual material	1 2 3 4

6) How will you integrate or use the information presented in this course?

_____
_____
_____
_____

7) What part of this course was most beneficial for you?

_____
_____
_____
_____

8) What part of this course was least beneficial for you?

_____
_____
_____
_____

9) Additional comments:

_____
_____
_____
_____

ADVANCED MEDICAL LIFE SUPPORT
INSTRUCTOR EVALUATION FORM

National Course #: _____ Course Location: _____

Country of Course Location: _____

Course Date(s): _____ Course Type: ☐ Provider ☐ Refresher ☐ Instructor ☐ Domestic ☐ Military

Healthcare Provider Level (Circle One)

Physician   Physician Assistant   Adv. Nurse Practitioner   Registered Nurse   EMT-Basic
    Paramedic   Other: _____

Lecture Topic: _____ Teaching/Testing Station: _____

Please rate the following aspects of the presenter and his or her presentation.
The following scale will be used:

1—Excellent
2—Good
3—Fair
4—Adequate

1) Presenter's ability to keep the audience's attention   1 2 3 4

2) Presenter's knowledge of lecture material   1 2 3 4

3) Presenter's ability to maintain the time schedule   1 2 3 4

4) Presenter's ability to integrate course material with practical application   1 2 3 4

5) Presenter's use of the audiovisual material   1 2 3 4

6) How will you integrate or use the information presented in this lecture?

_____
_____
_____
_____

7) What part of this lecture was most beneficial for you?

_____
_____
_____
_____

8) What part of this lecture was least beneficial for you?

_____
_____
_____
_____

9) Additional comments:

_____
_____
_____
_____

Advanced Medical Life Support
Instructor—Candidate Monitoring Form

Instructor-Candidate Name: _____

Provider Course Date: _____ Instructor Course Date: _____

Affiliate Faculty Monitor Name: _____

Lecture	Satisfactory	Unsatisfactory
Presents lecture in a logical, concise, sequential fashion		
Is familiar with the A/V slide content		
Emphasizes critical thinking skills and the field thinking process in the lecture		
Emphasizes "what's different" when comparing pathophysiology, signs, and symptoms on tables within the lecture. For example: auscultating breath sounds in determining causes of shock		
Maintains the participants' attention: — Varies pace, uses clear transitions — Uses questions appropriately — Has good voice, eye contact, and gestures — Moves purposefully — Does not read — Uses correct vocabulary and pronunciation		
Summarizes important points in the lecture and upon conclusion		
Uses appropriate examples to illustrate important points		
Answers questions in a supportive manner		
Completes the lecture on time		

Comments on lecture presentation: _____

_____

_____

_____

Instructor Attitude and Role	Satisfactory	Unsatisfactory
Attends faculty meetings		
Attends other lectures within the course		
Enhances the quality of the course		
Demonstrates support for the AMLS program		

Comments: _____

_____

_____

_____

Instructor-Candidate Name: _____

Provider Course Date: _____ Instructor Course Date: _____

Affiliate Faculty Monitor Name: _____

Group Case Scenario Stations	Satisfactory	Unsatisfactory
Prepares scenario's patient appropriately		
Presents scenario clearly and concisely		
Organizes equipment appropriately		
Allows team leader and team interaction to proceed without assistance		
Enhances critical thinking/field thinking process by intermittently asking about: — Initial impression and differential diagnoses — Initial plan — Initial assessment and resuscitation vs. gathering history first — Re-evaluation of impression and plan		
Allows team to lead discussion of each case and the processes used to manage the patient		
Summarizes topic of scenario and important points from lecture		

Comments on scenario presentation: _____

_____

_____

_____

Recommendation:

☐ Satisfactory

☐ Unsatisfactory. I recommend remediation and re-monitoring for possible future role
as an AMLS Instructor.

☐ Unsatisfactory. I recommend that this Candidate not be allowed to proceed as an AMLS Instructor.

Signature of Affiliate Faculty Monitor: _____ Date: _____

Date sent to AMLS Office: _____

Copy in File: _____

ADVANCED MEDICAL LIFE SUPPORT
PARTICIPANT FINAL EVALUATION FORM

Team Leader: _____ Scenario Number: _____

Evaluator: _____ Beginning Time: _____ Ending Time: _____

Task	Completed YES	Completed NO	Comments Regarding Deficiencies
Scene Safety			
Initial Impression			
Initial Assessment			
Mental Status			
Airway			
Breathing			
Circulation			
Disability/Perfusion			
Focused History (SAMPLE)			
Signs and Symptoms			
Allergies			
Medications			
Past Medical History			
Last Oral Intake			
Events Preceding			
OPQRST			
Onset			
Palliation/Provocation			
Quality			
Radiation			
Severity			
Time			
Vital Signs			
Respirations			
Pulse			
Blood Pressure			
Temperature			
Pulse Oximetry			
Focused Physical Exam			
Differential Diagnosis			
Appropriate Treatment			

Critical Criteria

The following areas have been identified as critical criteria. As such, if any item below is checked, the participant needs to repeat the station. Please document any rationale concerning the area checked in the notation section below.

☐ Body substance isolation not performed

☐ Scene was not determined to be safe

☐ Initial assessment not performed or performed in an inadequate manner

☐ Failure to adequately maintain Airway, Breathing, or Circulation at any time throughout the scenario

☐ Inability to establish stability vs. instability/life threat vs. non-life threat

☐ Focused history not performed or performed before initiation of life-saving measures

☐ Inappropriate treatment performed

☐ Appropriate treatment performed but in an untimely fashion

☐ Failure to complete the assessment in a timely manner

Additional Comments: _____

_____

_____

ADVANCED MEDICAL LIFE SUPPORT
PARTICIPANT EXAM ANSWER SHEET

Participant Name: _____ Date: _____ Score: _____

National Course #: _____ Course Location: _____

Country of Course Location: _____ ☐ Domestic ☐ Military

Circle and Mark One: BLS or ALS Pretest _____   BLS or ALS Post-test I _____   BLS or ALS Post-test II _____

1.	A	B	C	D
2.	A	B	C	D
3.	A	B	C	D
4.	A	B	C	D
5.	A	B	C	D
6.	A	B	C	D
7.	A	B	C	D
8.	A	B	C	D
9.	A	B	C	D
10.	A	B	C	D
11.	A	B	C	D
12.	A	B	C	D
13.	A	B	C	D
14.	A	B	C	D
15.	A	B	C	D
16.	A	B	C	D
17.	A	B	C	D
18.	A	B	C	D
19.	A	B	C	D
20.	A	B	C	D
21.	A	B	C	D
22.	A	B	C	D
23.	A	B	C	D
24.	A	B	C	D
25.	A	B	C	D

26.	A	B	C	D
27.	A	B	C	D
28.	A	B	C	D
29.	A	B	C	D
30.	A	B	C	D
31.	A	B	C	D
32.	A	B	C	D
33.	A	B	C	D
34.	A	B	C	D
35.	A	B	C	D
36.	A	B	C	D
37.	A	B	C	D
38.	A	B	C	D
39.	A	B	C	D
40.	A	B	C	D
41.	A	B	C	D
42.	A	B	C	D
43.	A	B	C	D
44.	A	B	C	D
45.	A	B	C	D
46.	A	B	C	D
47.	A	B	C	D
48.	A	B	C	D
49.	A	B	C	D
50.	A	B	C	D

ADVANCED MEDICAL LIFE SUPPORT
PROVIDER COURSE EVALUATION SUMMARY SHEET

National Course #: _____   Course Location: _____

Country of Course Location: _____

Course Date(s): _____   Course Type: ☐ Provider ☐ Refresher ☐ Instructor ☐ Domestic ☐ Military

Healthcare Provider Level (Circle One)

Physician   Physician Assistant   Adv. Nurse Practitioner   Registered Nurse   EMT-Basic
    Paramedic   Other: _____

Please rate the following lecture presentations:

Lecture Presentation	Extremely Useful	Very Useful	Fairly Useful	Not Useful	
Assessment of the Medical Patient					
Airway Management					
Hypoperfusion					
Dyspnea/Respiratory Failure					
Chest Pain					
Altered Mental Status					
Abdominal Pain/GI Bleed					

Comments: _____

_____

_____

_____

Teaching Group Scenarios	Extremely Useful	Very Useful	Fairly Useful	Not Useful	Not Applicable
Assessment of the Medical Patient					
Airway Management					
Hypoperfusion					
Dyspnea/Respiratory Failure					
Chest Pain					
Altered Mental Status					
Abdominal Pain/GI Bleed					

Comments: _____

_____

_____

_____

Evaluation Stations	Extremely Useful	Very Useful	Fairly Useful	Not Useful	Not Applicable
Scenarios					
Written Evaluation					

Where you informed about NAEMT and the benefits of membership? ☐ Yes ☐ No

Was the entire program well organized? ☐ Yes ☐ No

Comments: _____

_____

_____

_____

• Must be given to affiliate faculty and state coordinator.

ADVANCED MEDICAL LIFE SUPPORT COURSE ROSTER

National Course #: _____   State Course #: _____   Course Date: _____

Location/sponsor: _____

City, State, Zip: _____

LEVEL OF COURSE:
Advanced Provider (AP)
Combined Provider (CP)
Instructor (I)
Advanced Refresher (AR)
Combined Refresher (CR)

#	Student Name	Student Address	Phone Number	NAEMT Member (Y or N)	Course Level	Status Pass or Fail
1						
2						
3						
4						
5						
6						
7						
8						
9						
10						
11						
12						
13						
14						
15						

Advanced Medical Life Support Course Roster (Continued)

#	Student Name	Student Address	Phone Number	NAEMT Member (Y or N)	Course Level	Status Pass or Fail
16						
17						
18						
19						
20						
21						
22						
23						
24						
25						
26						
27						
28						
29						
30						
31						
32						
33						

This **AMLS** course was conducted as prescribed by the NAEMT/AMLS Program.

Course Coordinator

Course Medical Director

Affiliate Faculty (if present)

NAEMT

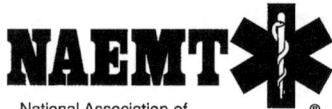

National Association of
Emergency Medical Technicians
P.O. Box 1400
Clinton, MS 39060-1400
1-800-34-NAEMT

Educational Program

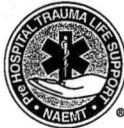

Participant Registration Form

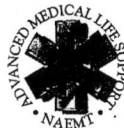

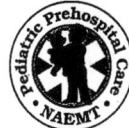

Participant

Please complete the following with a no. 2 pencil. This information is necessary to record your successful participation in this course and maintain records to verify your continuing education credit.

Are You Currently an NAEMT Member?   YES ☐   NO ☐

FIRST NAME   M.I.   LAST NAME   TITLE

ORGANIZATION

ADDRESS 1   ADDRESS 2

CITY   STATE/PRV   POSTAL CODE   COUNTRY

TELEPHONE 1   TELEPHONE 2   FAX

EMAIL ADDRESS   DATE OF BIRTH
M M D D Y Y
FEMALE ☐
MALE ☐

NATIONAL REGISTRY NO.   EXPIRATION DATE   STATE/PRV. CERT./ LIC. NO.   STATE/PRV.   EXPIRATION DATE
M M D D Y Y   M M D D Y Y

MILITARY IDENTIFICATION NO.

1st RESPONDER ☐   EMT-B ☐   EMT-I ☐
EMT-P ☐   PA ☐   RN ☐   MD ☐   OTHER ☐

Have you participated in an NAEMT Ed. program prior to this course? YES ☐   NO ☐

If you are not a member of NAEMT, you will be given a 1-year membership to NAEMT free and without obligation for your participation in this NAEMT educational program.

☐ **Check here if you do not wish to have your membership data released as part of our mailing list.**

Pre-test SCORE	FINAL SCORE	PASS / FAIL
		☐ ☐

To Be Completed By Instructors and Course Coordinators Only   *Instructors and Coordinators: please complete the following information with signatures before copying and distributing this form to course participants. Please see instructions on back of this form.*

Type of Course
AMLS ☐
PHTLS ☐
PPC ☐

National Course No.
☐☐ - ☐☐☐☐ - ☐☐

Course Dates
month   day   year   month   day   year
start ☐☐ / ☐☐ / ☐☐   end ☐☐ / ☐☐ / ☐☐

Course Site
Course Site No.

Course Coordinator
FIRST NAME   LAST NAME

Course Location
ORGANIZATION   CITY   STATE/ PROV.   COUNTRY

Course Coordinator Signature _____   Affiliate Faculty Signature _____

Medical Director Signature _____   Affiliate Faculty Signature _____

ADVANCED MEDICAL LIFE SUPPORT
INSTRUCTOR ROSTER

National Course #: _____ Course Location: _____

Country of Course Location: _____

Course Date(s): _____ Course Coordinator: _____

Course Type: ☐ Provider ☐ Refresher ☐ Instructor ☐ Domestic ☐ Military

Instructor Name Check ☐ if being monitored	E-Mail Address	Postal Address	Daytime Phone Number	AMLS Recognized Instructor	
☐				Y	N
☐				Y	N
☐				Y	N
☐				Y	N
☐				Y	N
☐				Y	N
☐				Y	N
☐				Y	N
☐				Y	N
☐				Y	N
☐				Y	N

• Must be given to state coordinator.

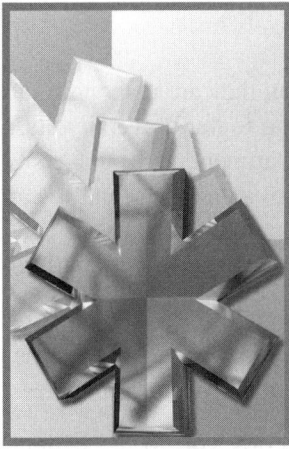

IV. CASE SCENARIOS FOR THE PROVIDER COURSE

ASSESSMENT OF THE MEDICAL PATIENT

▶ ASSESSMENT OF THE MEDICAL PATIENT: SCENARIO 1

Requirements: One instructor and one patient for every five participants.

Prerequisite: Read Chapter 1, "Assessment of the Medical Patient" and Chapter 11, "Syncope."

Equipment: One table and chair for the patient to use; jump kit with oxygen supplies. (NC, NRM, aerosol mask, PPV device, intubation equipment), stethoscope, blood pressure (BP) cuff, cardiac monitor, pulse oximeter, and medication kit with associated medications.

Instructor: Your role is vital because you must act as the coordinator of the station and also interact in the scenario. Before the participant arrives at the station, please review the scenario with your patient. Use moulage make-up to simulate pale skin.

Patient: One female patient. As the patient, you will be required to play the role of a 22-year-old female who is experiencing a severe headache. You will be awake and alert. Please read the scenario to familiarize yourself with the information.

Instructions

Hi, my name is _____, and I will be the instructor for this station. This is a hands-on patient assessment station. You will be given information concerning a patient experiencing a medical crisis. You will have all the necessary equipment you need to manage the patient in this station. Please look over the equipment before we go any further. You will be provided with pertinent information only when you ask the appropriate question. For any hands-on procedure, such as auscultation of a blood pressure or breath sounds or taking a pulse, select the appropriate equipment needed (if any) and use the equipment in the manner that it would be used on a patient. I will then give you the relevant clinical data. For example, you must select, place, and begin inflation of the BP cuff before the blood pressure is given to you. I will not answer questions in place of the patient. Therefore, it is imperative that you interact with your patient. Please verbalize to me any signs or symptoms that you find so that I will know you are cognizant of the patient and the patient's clinical appearance.

Scenario

It is a rainy spring morning. Advise the participants that they are responding to a call for a 22-year-old female who was preparing to go to her university class and developed a severe headache. The patient is in her apartment on the university campus. If the participants are nurses or in-hospital providers, the scenario can be modified to the medical environment—such as a patient in the emergency room triage waiting room. The participant should use the assessment taught in this course.

Initial Impression: 22-year-old female lying on her side on the couch in her basement apartment. She appears restless and agitated.

Scene Size-up/General Impression: A roommate escorts you to the patient. The scene is safe for entry and exit. No injury is apparent on brief visual exam.

Initial Assessment:
> *Mental Status*—Alert, Verbal, Pain, Unresponsive (AVPU) A&O × 3. Patient is able to answer questions appropriately, but frowns, closes eyes, and speaks very softly.

> *Airway*—Clear and patent, no evidence of injury, no C-spine precautions deemed necessary.

> *Breathing*—Shallow with equal rise of chest bilaterally. Pattern is regular and lungs clear.

> *Circulation*—Strong, rapid, irregular radial pulse. No external bleeding.

> *Disability/Perfusion*—Skin is cool, pale, and dry. Pupils, Equal, Round, Reactive to Light (PERRL).

> *Capillary Refill*—Less than 2 seconds. Patient can move all four extremities with equal strength.

> *Distal Pulses*—Regular and strong.

Status after Initial Assessment: Not life threatening, potentially unstable.

Possible Differential (Field) Diagnoses: Stroke, subdural hematoma, subarachnoid hemorrhage, endocrine emergency, carbon monoxide/toxic exposure, meningitis/encephalitis, migraine, cluster or tension headache. Encourage participants to respond and offer thoughts on other possibilities.

Initial Management Priorities: Oxygen at 4 lpm via nasal cannula, pulse oximetry, cardiac monitor, IV therapy

Focused History (SAMPLE):
> *Signs and Symptoms*—Patient laying recumbent. Patient is A&O × 3 with pale, cool, dry skin. Patient complains of a severe headache.

> *Allergies*—Sulfa medications.

> *Medications*—None prescribed. Patient has taken 800 mg of Ibuprofen 30 minutes prior to your arrival. She has no relief of pain with the Ibuprofen.

> *Past Medical History*—No chest pain or difficulty breathing. No known cardiac or respiratory problems. The patient has no history of headaches. She is not a diabetic. And has no history of recent illness.

Last Oral Intake—She attended a wine and cheese party the night before. She has had coffee and cereal for breakfast.

Events Preceding—The patient woke with a dull headache. The patient felt nauseous and sensitive to light upon waking this morning. She states the headache has increased in intensity.

OPQRST:

Onset—One hour prior to your arrival.

Palliation/Provocation—Unable to find a position of comfort. She complains of light and sound sensitivity. The pain increases with movement.

Quality—Throbbing and localized in the lower occipital area.

Radiation—Not relevant.

Severity—She states this is the worst headache she has ever had. The patient rates it a 10 on a 0–10 scale.

Time/Duration—One hour.

Vital Signs:

Respirations—18, regular and equal in symmetry

Pulse—Radial 120 bpm, rapid and strong

Blood Pressure—132/90

Temperature—98.6°F (37°C)

Pulse Oximetry—97%

Blood Glucose Level—98 mg/dl (5.4 mmol/L)

Focused Physical Exam (Focused Medical Assessment): Rapid head-to-toe is unremarkable. There is no sign of trauma. Neurological exam reveals no facial droop, no abnormal extraoccular movement, no nuchal rigidity, no hemiplegia. Strong bilateral strength in all four extremities.

Differential/Field Diagnosis: Migraine headache, ICH, increased ICP from pseudotumor, hydrocephalus. Potential contributing factors may be red wine, toxic fumes in basement apartment, or increased stress of course work.

Management:

1) Nasal cannula at 4 lpm.

2) IV access with 0.9% normal saline.

3) Cardiac monitor—Sinus tachycardia with occasional PACs.

4) Blood glucose level.

5) Transport in position of comfort with no cabin lights.

Detailed Physical Exam: En route to appropriate facility if time permits.

Ongoing Assessment: There is no change in patient's condition during transport.

Critical Actions:

1) Monitor airway because patient is a risk for vomiting.

2) Assess for injury and use C-spine precautions if necessary.

3) Maintain hemodynamic stability with blood pressure between 70–100 mmHg.

4) Assess for underlying life-threatening etiology for this headache episode.

5) Consider an analgesic and/or anti-emetic.

Teaching Points

1) There are numerous causes and etiologies for headaches:

   a) Hypertensive crisis (diastolic of at least 120 mmHg)

   b) Intracranial hemorrhage, tumors

   c) Pseudotumor cerebri or hydrocephalus

   d) Meningitis/encephalitis

   e) Fever

   f) Medications (oral contraceptives and nitrates)

   g) Emotional crisis, stress

   h) Toxic exposure (carbon monoxide, cyanide poisoning)

   i) Hypo/hyperglycemia with unusual behavior; BGL less than 50 mg/dl without signs and symptoms or BGL less than 60 mg/dl with signs and symptoms is considered hypoglycemic.

   j) Migraines

   k) A history of a sudden onset, rather than intensity, of pain is a best indicator of vascular etiology.

2) Migraine headaches have a tendency to be recurrent and primarily in female patients less than 30 years of age. Typical pain is unilateral throbbing with accompanying nausea and vomiting. Light (photophobia) and sound (sonophobia) sensitivity is common. Auras are often noted prior to a classic migraine. Headache pain is subjective and not a reliable indicator of severity. Migraine headaches are associated with an initial vasoconstriction of intracranial arteries which cause ischemia. The ischemia results in a vasaodilatory effect. Serotonin and dopamine levels play a role in the pathophysiology of these type of headaches. Stimulating dopamine receptors results in the common nausea, vomiting, and agitation. Serotonin can be used to reduce the symptoms of a migraine. About 10% have focal neurologic deficits.

3) An organized approach and thorough patient history will assist in ruling out possible causes. Cognitive and neurological deficits should be identified and managed as having a serious etiology.

Evaluation

1) *Excellent:* The participants' evaluation of the patient followed set format: initial assessment, focused history (SAMPLE, OPQRST) in an efficient manner. The participants displayed a thorough knowledge of the patient's condition, performed the exam and management in an organized manner, and demonstrated an excellent overall performance.

2) *Good:* The participants' evaluation of the patient followed set format: initial assessment, focused history (SAMPLE, OPQRST) in an acceptable manner with only minor deviation. The participants displayed an above-average knowledge of the patient's condition, performed the exam and management of the patient's condition, and demonstrated an above-average performance.

3) *Fair:* The participants' evaluation of the patient deviated from the set format without causing any further injury to the patient. The participants displayed an average or basic knowledge of the patient's condition and performed an adequate exam and management of the patient's condition.

4) *Inadequate:* The participants' evaluation of the patient deviated significantly from the set format, or the participants' actions endangered the patient's life or significantly exacerbated the condition.

► ASSESSMENT OF THE MEDICAL PATIENT: SCENARIO 2

Requirements: One instructor and one patient for every five participants.

Prerequisite: Read Chapter 1, "Assessment of the Medical Patient" and Chapter 11, "Syncope."

Equipment: One table and chair for the patient to use; jump kit with oxygen supplies (NC, NRM, aerosol mask, PPV device, intubation equipment), stethoscope, BP cuff, cardiac monitor, pulse oximeter, and medication kit with associated medications.

Instructor: Your role is vital because you must act as the coordinator of the station and also interact in the scenario. Before the participant arrives at the station, please review the scenario with your patient. Spray the patient's arms with a fine mist of cool water to simulate cool, clammy skin. Use moulage make-up to simulate skin color.

Patient: One male (or female) patient. As the patient, you will be required to play the role of a 42-year-old male who is experiencing a fever with vomiting. You will be awake and alert. Please read the scenario to familiarize yourself with the information.

Instructions

Hi, my name is _____, and I will be the instructor for this station. This is a hands-on patient assessment station. You will be given information concerning a patient experiencing a medical crisis. You will have all the necessary equipment you need to manage the patient in this station. Please look over the equipment before we go any further. You will be provided with pertinent information only when you ask the appropriate question. For any hands-on procedure, such as auscultation of a blood pressure or breath sounds or taking a pulse, select the appropriate equipment needed (if any) and use the equipment in the manner that it would be used on a patient. I will then give you the relevant clinical data. For example, you must select, place, and begin inflation of the BP cuff before the blood pressure is given to you. I will not answer questions in place of the patient. Therefore, it is imperative that you interact with your patient. Please verbalize to me any signs or symptoms that you find so that I will know you are cognizant of the patient and the patient's clinical appearance.

Scenario

Advise the participants that it is 1300 hours and they are responding to a call for a 42-year-old male who is complaining of feeling ill with a fever, extremity pain, and vomiting. He is at his one-level residence. If the participants are nurses or in-hospital providers, the scenario can be modified to the medical environment—such as a patient admitted to Room 5 in the emergency room. The participant should use the assessment taught in this course.

Initial Impression: 42-year-old male (or female) is grimacing with head and neck pain sitting in a chair in the living room of his residence. There is a waste can with 100 cc of vomit beside the chair.

Scene Size-up/General Impression: His wife escorts you to the patient. The scene is safe for entry and exit. No injury is apparent on brief visual exam.

Initial Assessment:

Mental Status—AVPU: A&O × 3. Patient is able to answer questions appropriately.

Airway—Clear and patent, no evidence of injury, no C-spine precautions deemed necessary.

Breathing—Deep and rapid with equal rise of chest bilaterally. Lungs are clear.

Circulation—Weak, rapid, thready radial pulse. No external bleeding.

Disability/Perfusion: Skin is hot, dry, and flushed. Pupils are equal and sluggish. Capillary Refill: Less than 2 seconds. Patient has pain with flexion and extension of extremities. Distal pulses regular and weak.

Status after Initial Assessment: Not life threatening, potentially unstable.

Possible Differential (Field) Diagnoses: Hyperglycemia diabetic ketocidosis (DKA) secondary to infection, intracranial infection, and Lyme disease. Painful extremities may indicate myositis, septic joint, or immune-mediated disease. Encourage participants to respond and offer thoughts on other possibilities.

Initial Management Priorities: Oxygen via non-rebreather mask, pulse oximetry, cardiac monitor, IV therapy.

Focused History (SAMPLE):

Signs and Symptoms—Patient slumped in chair after episode of vomiting. Patient is A&O × 3, with hot, dry, flushed skin. Patient has experienced lightheadedness and complaines of a severe headache.

Allergies—no known allergies (NKA)

Medications—Zovirax (acyclovir) ointment 5% prn. Patient has taken over-the-counter (OTC) sinus medication for a sinus infection which has lasted one week. OTC medications have not resolved the sinus infection.

Past Medical History—Herpes Simplex which is localized to the face. No palpitations, chest pain, or difficulty breathing. No known cardiac or respiratory problems. The patient has never had a syncopal episode. No history of stroke, headaches, or diabetes.

Last Oral Intake—Oatmeal and juice for a late breakfast.

Events Preceding—Patient has had a fever for several days along with a sinus infection. He has felt lightheaded today, but has not had a syncopal episode. He has developed a severe headache which has worsened since this morning.

OPQRST:

Onset—One hour prior to your arrival. Patient's headache, vomiting, and fever are worsening with time, while patient is at rest.

Palliation/Provocation—No relief from OTC sinus medication or rest.

Quality—Throbbing, persistent headache, extremity pain, and nausea severe and worsening with time.

Radiation—Not relevant.

Severity—Rates headache and extremity pain a 9 on a 0–10 scale.

Time/Duration—One hour.

Vital Signs:

Respirations—22, deep and rapid, and equal in symmetry

Pulse—Radial 132 bpm, weak and rapid

Blood Pressure—134/86

Temperature—102°F (38.8°C)

Pulse Oximetry—97%

Blood Glucose Level—86 mg/dl (4.7 mmol/L)

Focused Physical Exam (Focused Medical Assessment): Focused physical exam reveals extremity pain and neck pain with flexion and extension movement. Neurological exam reveals patient is visually sensitive to light. There is no facial droop or slurred speech. Patient has nuchal rigidity and a positive Kernig's sign.

Differential/Field Diagnosis: Meningitis/abscess/cavernous sinus thrombosis from sinus infection; encephalitis related to herpes simplex viral infection; subarachnoid/intracranial hemorrhage are all probable.

Management:
1) Non-rebreather at 15 lpm to maintain adequate oxygen saturation
2) IV access with 0.9% normal saline
3) Cardiac monitor—sinus tachycardia with no ectopy
4) Blood glucose level
5) Transport in position of comfort

Detailed Physical Exam: En route to appropriate facility if time permits.

Ongoing Assessment: There is no change in patient's condition during transport.

Critical Actions:
1) Maintain airway and be prepared to suction related to vomiting and risk for syncope.
2) Assess for injury and use C-spine precautions if necessary.
3) Maintain hemodynamic stability with systolic blood pressure greater than 90 mmHg.
4) Assess for underlying life-threatening etiology for intracranial infection.
5) Monitor neurological status closely; be ready for decrease in mental status.

Teaching Points

1) There are numerous causes and etiologies for intracranial infections. Identifying a definitive cause is difficult in the prehospital environment.

   a) Meningitis and encephalitis are difficult to differentiate between because the signs and symptoms are similar.

   b) Meningitis can be caused by a fungus, virus, bacteria, or any pathogen that migrates to the meningeal membranes. Encephalitis is most commonly caused by viral pathogens.

   c) Increased intracranial pressure results from inflammation of the meningeal layers.

d) Alterations in mentation and seizure activity indicate significant infection and inflammation to the meninges.

e) Nuchal rigidity and neck stiffness are the result of inflammation of the meninges over the spinal cord. Brudzinski and Kernig's signs are indications of meningeal irritation.

f) Viral infections, such as herpes and rabies, are often etiologies that result in encephalitis.

g) Coma results if both cerebral hemispheres and the reticular activating system (RAS) are involved.

h) A history of associated fever, malaise, decline in mentation, persistent headache, vision disturbances, seizure activity, hemiparesis, and hemiplegia indicate a cranial infection that is a life threat.

2) An organized approach and thorough patient history will assist in ruling out possible causes.

Evaluation

1) *Excellent:* The participant's evaluation of the patient followed set format: initial assessment, focused history (SAMPLE, OPQRST) in an efficient manner. The participant displayed a thorough knowledge of the patient's condition, performed the exam and management in an organized manner, and demonstrated an excellent overall performance.

2) *Good:* The participant's evaluation of the patient followed set format: initial assessment, focused history (SAMPLE, OPQRST) in an acceptable manner with only minor deviation. The participant displayed an above-average knowledge of the patient's condition, performed the exam and management of the patient's condition, and demonstrated an above-average performance.

3) *Fair:* The participant's evaluation of the patient deviated from the set format without causing any further injury to the patient. The participant displayed an average or basic knowledge of the patient's condition and performed an adequate exam and management of the patient's condition.

4) *Inadequate:* The participant's evaluation of the patient deviated significantly from the set format, or the participant's actions endangered the patient's life or significantly exacerbated the condition.

▶ Assessment of the Medical Patient: Scenario 3

Requirements: One instructor and one patient for every five participants.

Prerequisite: Read Chapter 1, "Assessment of the Medical Patient" and Chapter 11, "Syncope."

Equipment: One table and chair for the patient to use; jump kit with oxygen supplies (NC, NRM, aerosol mask, PPV device, intubation equipment), stethoscope, BP cuff, cardiac monitor, pulse oximeter, and medication kit with associated medications.

Instructor: Your role is vital because you must act as the coordinator of the station and also interact in the scenario. Before the participant arrives at the station, please review the scenario with your patient. Spray the patient's arms with a fine mist of cool water to simulate cool, clammy skin. Use moulage make-up to simulate pale skin.

Patient: One male (or female) patient. As the patient, you will be required to play the role of a 62-year-old male who has experienced a syncopal episode. You will be awake and alert. Please read the scenario to familiarize yourself with the information.

Instructions

Hi, my name is _____, and I will be the instructor for this station. This is a hands-on patient assessment station. You will be given information concerning a patient experiencing a medical crisis. You will have all the necessary equipment you need to manage the patient in this station. Please look over the equipment before we go any further. You will be provided with pertinent information only when you ask the appropriate question. For any hands-on procedure, such as auscultation of a blood pressure or breath sounds or taking a pulse, select the appropriate equipment needed (if any) and use the equipment in the manner that it would be used on a patient. I will then give you the relevant clinical data. For example, you must select, place, and begin inflation of the BP cuff before the blood pressure is given to you. I will not answer questions in place of the patient. Therefore, it is imperative that you interact with your patient. Please verbalize to me any signs or symptoms that you find so that I will know you are cognizant of the patient and the patient's clinical appearance.

Scenario

It is a warm, humid afternoon in August. Advise the participants that they are responding to a call for a 62-year-old male who stood up to get refreshments and experienced what appears to be a syncopal episode. The patient was watching his grandson's Little League game. If the participants are nurses or in-hospital providers, the scenario can be modified to the medical environment—such as a patient in the emergency room (ER) waiting room collapsed while standing and is being escorted to triage. The participants should use the assessment taught in this course.

Initial Impression: 62-year-old male (or female) sitting in a lawn chair with legs elevated on a cooler. The patient is positioned at the baseball field sideline.

Scene Size-up/General Impression: Local police department escorts you to the patient. Crowd control is managed and the scene is safe for entry and exit.

No injury is apparent on brief visual exam. Family members surround patient and are helpful with the history of events. Watch out for foul balls!

Initial Assessment:

Mental Status—AVPU: A&O × 3. Patient is able to answer questions appropriately.

Airway—Clear and patent, no evidence of injury, no C-spine precautions deemed necessary.

Breathing—Unlabored, equal rise of chest bilaterally, regular pattern; lungs clear.

Circulation —Weak, rapid, thready radial pulse. No external bleeding.

Disability/Perfusion:
Skin is cool, pale, and moist. Pupils PERRL. Capillary refill less than 2 seconds. Patient can move all four extremities with equal strength. Distal pulses regular and weak.

Status after Initial Assessment:
Not life threatening, potentially unstable.

Possible Differential (Field) Diagnosis:
Transient Ischemic Attack, stroke, seizure, cardiovascular event (acute coronary syndrome; dysrhythmia), dehydration, vasovagal response, hypoglycemia, environmental emergency. Encourage participants to respond and offer thoughts on other possibilities.

Initial Management Priorities:
Oxygen at 4 lpm via nasal cannula, pulse oximetry, cardiac monitor, IV therapy.

Focused History (SAMPLE):

Signs and Symptoms—Elderly patient seated with legs elevated in warm environment. Patient is A&O × 3, with pale, cool, clammy skin. Patient has experienced a syncopal episode.

Allergies—Penicillin.

Medications—None prescribed. Patient does not take OTC medications, beta-blockers, nitrates, or diuretics.

Past Medical History—No palpitations, chest pain, or difficulty breathing. No known cardiac or respiratory problems. The patient has never had a syncopal episode. No history of stroke or diabetes.

Last Oral Intake—Light lunch and ice tea.

Events Preceding—Patient does not remember syncopal episode. He became syncopal when standing up to get refreshments.

OPQRST:

Onset—10 minutes prior to your arrival, when rising to get refreshments

Palliation/Provocation—Sitting down with legs elevated

Quality—Transient, quickly resolved

Radiation—Not relevant

Severity—Brief loss of consciousness, did not fall to ground

Time/Duration—Approximately 10 seconds

Vital Signs:

Respirations—18, regular and equal in symmetry

Pulse—Radial 128 bpm, weak and rapid and irregular

Blood Pressure—92/68

Temperature—98.6°F (37°C)

Cardiac Monitor—Reveals atrial fibrillation

Pulse Oximetry—97%

Blood Glucose Level—98 mg/dl (5.4 mmol/L)

Focused Physical Exam (Focused Medical Assessment): Rapid head-to-toe is unremarkable. Skin tenting is negative. Neurological exam reveals no facial droop, slurred speech, and strong bilateral strength in all four extremities. There is no positive tilt test. No pedal edema.

Differential/Field Diagnosis: Syncope related to new onset of atrial fibrillation in association with mild dehydration. Contributing factors may be dehydration and remaining sedentary for a long period of time.

Management:

1) Nasal cannula at 4 lpm.

2) IV access with 0.9% normal saline. Fluid bolus 200–500 ml.

3) Cardiac monitor—atrial fibrillation with no ectopy.

4) Blood glucose level.

5) Transport in recumbent position.

Detailed Physical Exam: En route to appropriate facility if time permits.

Ongoing Assessment: There is no change in patient's condition during transport.

Critical Actions:

1) Secure airway and suction as necessary.

2) Assess for injury and use C-spine precautions if necessary.

3) Maintain hemodynamic stability with blood pressure greater than 90 mmHg.

   a) Control ventricular rate if causing poor perfusion or symptoms of cardiac ischemia

   b) IV therapy as needed (assure no pulmonary edema)

4) Assess for underlying life-threatening etiology for syncopal episode.

Teaching Points

1) There are numerous causes and etiologies for syncope.

   a) Vasovagal syncope

   b) Orthostatic hypotension related to beta blockers, diuretics, fluid losses, bleeding (may be internal)

   c) Bradyarrhythmias, such as AV nodal block, sick sinus syndrome, sinus bradycardia, or sinus arrest

   d) Tachyarrhythmias (VT, SVT, rapid AF), especially at a rate greater than 180 bpm

   e) Emotional crisis

f) Pain

g) Hypo/hyperglycemia with unusual behavior; BGL less than 50 mg/dl without signs and symptoms or BGL less than 60 mg/dl with signs and symptoms is considered hypoglycemic.

h) Stroke or other intracranial condition

2) An organized approach and thorough patient history will assist in ruling out possible causes.

Evaluation

1) *Excellent:* The participant's evaluation of the patient followed set format: initial assessment, focused history (SAMPLE, OPQRST) in an efficient manner. The participant displayed a thorough knowledge of the patient's condition, performed the exam and management in an organized manner, and demonstrated an excellent overall performance.

2) *Good:* The participant's evaluation of the patient followed set format: initial assessment, focused history (SAMPLE, OPQRST) in an acceptable manner with only minor deviation. The participant displayed an above-average knowledge of the patient's condition, performed the exam and management of the patient's condition, and demonstrated an above-average performance.

3) *Fair:* The participant's evaluation of the patient deviated from the set format without causing any further injury to the patient. The participant displayed an average or basic knowledge of the patient's condition and performed an adequate exam and management of the patient's condition.

4) *Inadequate:* The participant's evaluation of the patient deviated significantly from the set format, or the participant's actions endangered the patient's life or significantly exacerbated the condition.

▶ ASSESSMENT OF THE MEDICAL PATIENT: SCENARIO 4

Requirements: One instructor and one patient for every five participants.

Prerequisites: Read Chapter 1, "Assessment of the Medical Patient" and Chapter 12, "Headache, Nausea, and Vomiting."

Equipment: One table and chair for the patient to use; jump kit with oxygen supplies (NC, NRM, aerosol mask, PPV device, intubation equipment), stethoscope, BP cuff, cardiac monitor, pulse oximeter, and medication kit with assorted medications.

Instructor: Your role is vital because you must act as the coordinator of the station and also interact in the scenario. Before the participant arrives at the station, please review the scenario with your patient. Spray the patient's face and arms with a fine mist of cool water to simulate cool, clammy skin. Use moulage make-up to simulate pale skin.

Patient: One female patient. As the patient, you will be required to play the role of a 34-year-old female who has had nausea and vomiting for two days. You will be awake and alert. Please read the scenario to familiarize yourself with the information.

Instructions

Hi, my name is _____, and I will be the instructor for this station. This is a hands-on patient assessment station. You will be given information concerning a patient experiencing a medical crisis. You will have all the necessary equipment you need to manage the patient in this station. Please look over the equipment before we go any further. You will be provided with pertinent information only when you ask the appropriate question. For any hands-on procedure, such as auscultation of a blood pressure or breath sounds or taking a pulse, select the appropriate equipment needed (if any) and use the equipment in the manner that it would be used on a patient. I will then give you the relevant clinical data. For example, you must select, place, and begin inflation of the BP cuff before the blood pressure is given to you. I will not answer questions in place of the patient. Therefore, it is imperative that you interact with your patient. Please verbalize to me any signs or symptoms that you find so that I will know you are cognizant of the patient and the patient's clinical appearance.

Scenario

Advise the participants that they are asked to evaluate a 34-year-old female who has had nausea and vomiting for two days. The patient is lying on a couch in her living room. If the participants are nurses or in-hospital providers, the scenario can be modified to the medical environment—such as the patient is in ER Room 5. The participant should use the assessment taught in this course.

Initial Impression: 34-year-old female lying on a couch at residence. There is a bucket beside the couch with approximately 250 cc of vomit in it.

Scene Size-up/General Impression: Family members escort you to the patient. Family members do not speak English, but the patient does. There is easy access to the patient. No safety issues are noted. Patient is lying very still in lateral fetal position. No obvious signs of drug or alcohol use exist.

Initial Assessment:

Mental Status—AVPU: A&O × 3. Patient is able to answer questions appropriately.

Airway—No evidence of injury present. Airway clear and patent, no suction required.

Breathing—Unlabored, symmetrical chest rise; rate and rhythm regular; lungs clear.

Circulation—Bounding, rapid, and irregular radial pulse. No external bleeding noted.

Disability/Perfusion: Skin is cool, pale, and moist. Pupils PERRL. Capillary refill 4 seconds. Patient can move all extremities with equal strength.

Status after Initial Assessment: Not life threatening, potentially unstable. No evidence of aspiration.

Possible Differential (Field) Diagnosis: Sepsis, cerebral edema ICP, renal calculi, myocardial ischemia, diabetic ketoacidosis, uremia, toxicologic emergencies, ectopic pregnancy, intra-uterine pregnancy, other intra-abdominal emergencies (e.g., ruptured appendicitis, bowel obstruction, vertigo, labyrinthitis, cholecystitis, pancreatitis), ruptured esophagus (Booerhave's syndrome), acute gastroenteritis with dehydration.

Initial Management Priorities: Oxygen at 4 lpm via nasal cannula, pulse oximetry, cardiac monitor, IV therapy.

Focused History (SAMPLE):

Signs and Symptoms—Pale, cool, clammy skin; bounding, weak, irregular pulse; position of comfort lateral recumbent; no headache, stiff neck. Vomiting is not projectile.

Allergies—NKA.

Medications—Birth control, OTC anti-emetic.

Past Medical History—None other than vomiting last two days; no menses cycle problems; no risk of pregnancy.

Last Oral Intake—Unable to eat or drink last two days. Has not eaten at a restaurant this week.

Events Preceding—Woke out of sleep this morning with nausea and vomiting. Has been vomiting for two days without relief of OTC anti-emetic.

OPQRST:

Onset—Last two days.

Palliation/Provocation—Nothing makes it better. Vomiting not associated with food intake.

Quality—Cramping in abdomen prior to need for vomiting.

Radiation—Not relevant.

Severity—7 on a 0–10 scale.

Time/Duration—Infrequent vomiting episodes yesterday, more frequent today.

Vital Signs:

Respirations—24, regular and shallow, equal rise and fall of chest bilaterally

Pulse—Radial at 118 bpm, irregular and bounding

Blood Pressure—88/60

Temperature—101.2°F (38.8°C)

Pulse Oximetry—98%

Blood Glucose Level—80 mg/dl (4.4 mmol/L)

Focused Physical Exam (Focused Medical Assessment): Rapid head-to-toe is unremarkable. Skin tenting present. Neurological exam reveals strong bilateral strength in all four extremities. Pulses weak in lower extremities. No pedal edema. No bruising, ascites, distention, rigidity, or pulsating masses to abdominal area. No pain on palpation, no rebound tenderness.

Differential/Field Diagnoses: Nausea and vomiting with hypotension, electrolyte imbalance, metabolic alkalosis, dehydration.

Management:

1) Nasal cannula at 4 lpm.

2) IV access with 0.9% normal saline. May require additional boloses.

3) Cardiac monitor—sinus tachycardia with occasional PACs at a rate of 118.

4) Blood glucose level D_{50} if hypoglycemic.

5) Assessment of color, consistency, odor and amount of vomit.

6) Administration of anti-emetics

a) Compazine: 5–10 mg IM or IVP to block chemoreceptor trigger zone in vomit center of the brain (medulla)

b) Phenergan: 10–25 mg IM or IVP to compete with histamine for H1 receptor site in GI tract

7) Transport in position of comfort with reassessment of airway.

Detailed Physical Exam: En route to appropriate facility if time permits.

Ongoing Assessment: There is no change in patient's condition during transport. Patient does not experience any vomiting episodes while under your care.

Critical Actions:

1) Secure airway and suction if necessary.

2) Maintain hemodynamic stability with blood pressure greater than 90 mmHg.

3) Assess for underlying life-threatening etiology for persistent nausea and vomiting.

Teaching Points

1) There are numerous causes and etiologies for persistent nausea and vomiting.

a) Inner ear infections with vertigo (labyrinthitis).

b) If nausea is relieved after eating, it may be related to gastritis. If nausea is increased after eating, it may be associated with a peptic ulcer.

c) If vomiting is projectile, it may be associated with increased or elevated intracranial pressure.

d) Restlessness and blood in urine may indicate obstructive urinary tract (e.g., kidney stone) disease.

e) Blood in vomit-GI bleeding (esophageal varices, ulcer)

f) Duration and frequency of vomiting may precipitate dehydration.

g) Nausea and vomiting may be associated with AMI, DKA, new medication toxicity or hypersensitivity, drug overdose, hypertensive crisis, migraine headache, or ruptured ovarian cyst.

h) Bowel obstruction, pancreatitis, hepatitis, biliary disease, pyelonephritis are also concerns.

2) An organized approach and thorough patient history will assist in ruling out possible causes.

Evaluation

1) *Excellent:* The participant's evaluation of the patient followed set format: initial assessment, focused history (SAMPLE, OPQRST) in an efficient manner. The participant displayed a thorough knowledge of the patient's condition, performed the exam and management in an organized manner, and demonstrated an excellent overall performance.

2) *Good:* The participant's evaluation of the patient followed set format: initial assessment, focused history (SAMPLE, OPQRST) in an acceptable manner with only minor deviation. The participant displayed an above-average knowledge of the patient's condition, performed the exam and management of the patient's condition, and demonstrated an above-average performance.

3) *Fair:* The participant's evaluation of the patient deviated from the set format without causing any further injury to the patient. The participant displayed an average or basic knowledge of the patient's condition and performed an adequate exam and management of the patient's condition.

4) *Inadequate:* The participant's evaluation of the patient deviated significantly from the set format, or the participant's actions endangered the patient's life or significantly exacerbated the condition.

⊞ AIRWAY MANAGEMENT

▶ AIRWAY MANAGEMENT: SCENARIO 1

Requirements: One instructor and one manikin for every five participants.

Prerequisites: Read Chapter 2, "Airway Management, Ventilation, and Oxygen Therapy."

Airway (Optional) Scenarios: Equipment
Standard precautions equipment: gloves, face shield, mask, etc.

One adult airway manikin for every five participants with the following:
—Lubricant for manikin (according to manufacturer)
—Adult bag-valve-mask system
—Mouth-to-mask device for ventilation
—End-tidal CO_2 detector (colormetric)
—Esophageal detection device
—Capnography equipment (optional)
—Pulse oximeter and probe (optional)
—Cardiac monitor/defibrillator/pacer system (optional)
—Oxygen supplement appliances: non-rebreather mask, simple mask, etc. (optional)
—Stethoscope
—Various adult-sized oropharyngeal airways
—Various adult-sized nasopharyngeal airways
—Dual-lumen combination tube (CombiTube) with syringes and gastric tube or PtL device with syringes
—Laryngeal mask airway (LMA), COBRA PLA or King LTD with appropriate syringes (optional)
—Adult-sized (various) endotracheal tubes with syringes and stylets
—Scenario medication kit with various sedative and paralytic agents (optional)

Instructor: Your role is important because you act as the coordinator of the station, assembling and troubleshooting equipment, and act as the facilitator of the scenario presented. Before the participant arrives, arrange equipment, lubricate manikin, check laryngoscope, etc. Please read the scenarios to become familiar with the necessary responses. As the scenario is introduced to the participants involved, answer questions asked but do not offer more information than would be obvious in looking at a patient.

Instructions

Hi, my name is _____, and I will be the instructor for this station. This is a hands-on patient assessment station. You will be given information concerning a patient experiencing a medical crisis. You will have all the necessary equipment you need to manage the patient in this station. Please look over the equipment before we go any further. You will be provided with pertinent information only when you ask the appropriate question. For any hands-on procedure, such as auscultation of a blood pressure or breath sounds or taking a pulse, select the appropriate equipment needed (if any) and use the equipment in the manner that it would be used on a patient. I will then give you the relevant clinical data. For example, you must select, place, and begin inflation of the BP cuff before the blood pressure is given to you. I will not answer questions in place of the patient. Therefore, it is imperative that you interact with your patient. Please verbalize to me any signs or symptoms that you find so that I will know you are cognizant of the patient and the patient's clinical appearance.

Scenario

Advise the participants that they are responding to a local, small hospital to transport a medical patient to another facility with specialized resources. The participant should use the assessment taught in this course.

Initial Impression: 56-year-old female lying on the Emergency Department cart with eyes closed, pale, working hard to breathe, with tachypnea.

Possible Differential (Field) Diagnoses: Altered mental status, potential stroke vs. blood chemistry alteration vs. shock vs. respiratory ailment with hypoxia, etc.

Scene Size-up/General Impression: Scene is safe. No obvious trauma noted. This patient appears to weigh approximately 150 lbs (68 kg).

Initial Assessment:
 Mental Status—Responds to painful stimuli by pushing your hand away (localizes).

 Airway—No secretions visible. Swallows without effort spontaneously. Air is *moving.*

 Breathing—Respiratory effort labored with accessory muscle use and at an increased rate. Breath sounds are heard easily throughout fields without crackles.

 Circulation—Radial pulses palpable at 90 per minute. No verbal response. Does not follow commands.

Disability/Perfusion: Skin color is pale, warm, and dry. Glasgow Coma score of 7. Moves all extremities spontaneously.

Status after Initial Assessment: Unstable, potential life threat.

Possible Differential (Field) Diagnoses: CNS event (CVA, bleed, elevated ICP), sepsis, DKA, HHNKS, metabolic acidosis, PE.

Initial Management Priorities: NRM, cardiac monitor, pulse oximetry, IV therapy. Be prepared for BVM ventilation.

Focused History (SAMPLE):
 Signs and Symptoms—The nurse at the bedside relates that this 56-year-old was admitted to their ED this morning (2 hours ago) with decreased level of consciousness.

 Allergies—Codeine.

 Medications—Humulin insulin—regular and NPH; Acetylsalicylic Acid; Potassium; Furosemide; Digitalis; Nifedipine.

 Past Medical History—Diabetes, hypertension, heart disease.

 Last Oral Intake—Unknown—was found by a neighbor like this.

 Events Preceding—Patient lives on her own. Neighbor found her this morning on the couch in this state. Neighbor thought she was OK these past 2 days—not sure.

OPQRST:

Onset—Found 2 hours ago. Last seen up and about 2 days ago.

Palliation/Provocation—Patient not conversant.

Quality—Patient not conversant.

Radiation—Not applicable.

Severity—Not applicable.

Time/Duration—Found 2 hours ago; unknown duration. Patient's apartment seemed slightly messy—"not like her," according to neighbor.

Vital Signs:

Respirations—30, deep

Pulse—90 bpm at the radius

Blood Pressure—150/100

Temperature—101°F (38.3°C)

Pulse Oximetry—92% on room air, 95% with oxygen via non-rebreather

Blood Glucose Level—800 mg/dl (44.0 mmol/L) on admission

Focused Physical Exam (Focused Medical Assessment): Head-to-toe exam reveals a slightly obese female with distended abdomen who is working hard to breathe. No obvious trauma, no open wounds, no obvious signs of infection. Sinus tachycardia on lead 2. Arterial blood gases (ABGs) in the ED show pH of 7.10, pCO_2 of 15, pO_2 of 90, HCO_3 −12 with base excess of −6.

Differential/Field Diagnosis: Diabetic ketoacidosis with low level of consciousness.

Management:

1) Due to patient's low level of consciousness, definitive airway management for airway protection should be performed prior to commencing transfer.

   a) High-flow oxygen is being administered.

   b) Two IVs should be established at a wide open rate for at least 2 liters.

   c) All monitoring equipment applied.

   d) RSI protocol should be followed. (Participant should check potassium level if using succinylcholine.)

   e) Appropriately sized endotracheal tube inserted, assessed for placement using two techniques, and secured at the proper depth.

   f) Participant should discuss RSI failed intubation protocols. NOTE: If EMT-Bs are participating in these groups, they are integral in assisting in RSI procedures. Make sure they understand their role in providing Sellick's maneuver, BVM ventilation, etc.

2) Discuss appropriate respiratory assessment during transport.

3) Continue monitoring and medication administration for assisted respiration during transport.

4) Discuss proper ventilation rate and depth.

Detailed Physical Exam: En route to appropriate facility as time permits.

Ongoing Assessment: Continue evaluation of respiratory effort and level of consciousness.

Critical Actions:

1) Recognize the potential for airway and ventilation problems during the transfer of a patient with a diminished Glasgow Coma score.

2) Proper assessment for and demonstration of the generic protocol for medication-assisted intubation techniques.

3) Management of the intubated patient with positive pressure ventilation in regards to proper monitoring techniques, continued sedation and paralytic administration, and ventilation therapy.

Teaching Points

1) For a complicated medical patient such as described in this case, an advanced level of EMS care should be provided. This advanced care should include good assessment and management skills for airway and ventilation therapy.

2) The groups should discuss alternative airway securement options if RSI is not available. They should also discuss what options the Emergency medical services (EMS) crews have if the local physician performs RSI and expects them to continue sedation and paralytic administration without having appropriate protocols.

3) There are literally hundreds of variances in how to perform RSI. Each advanced EMS crew should follow their medical director's guidance in this procedure and understand every nuance of their protocol.

4) The pathophysiology involved in this case includes an insulin-dependent diabetic in diabetic ketoacidosis (DKA). The instructor should discuss causes of DKA, common clinical findings, and treatment. The case should create discussion on the possibility of this patient having hyperkalemia and the consequences of that within certain RSI protocols with options available (e.g., succinylcholine should be avoided in cases with hyperkalemia).

Evaluation

1) *Excellent:* The participants evaluated and recognized the need for a more secure airway prior to transport. They worked as a team to complete the medical assessment of the patient including SAMPLE, OPQRST, and a focused exam. They assessed for complications of intubation and use of the RSI procedure; they had a back-up plan in place for the potential for failed RSI. They demonstrated good skills and discussed appropriate monitoring and ventilation technique.

2) *Good:* The group evaluated the patient using the standard medical assessment format and recognized the patient with a low level of consciousness with potential for airway compromise. They displayed an above-average knowledge of advanced airway management and alternatives for this patient's condition. They were able to perform the skills of airway

management and discussed with the instructor the steps in RSI and complications.

3) *Fair:* The group evaluated the patient with some assistance from the instructor. They recognized the need for advanced airway management but had to be taught how to perform these procedures. They followed the lead of the instructor in assessing for complications of intubation and RSI. They could provide basic airway and ventilation skills with assistance in pathophysiology of this case.

4) *Inadequate:* The entire station had to be taught by the instructor. The group was unable to provide a medical assessment, unable to identify pathophysiology, and unable to appropriately manage the basics without being led by the instructor.

▶ AIRWAY MANAGEMENT: SCENARIO 2

Requirements: One instructor and one manikin for every five participants.

Prerequisites: Read Chapter 2, "Airway Management, Ventilation, and Oxygen Therapy."

Airway (Optional) Scenarios: Equipment
Standard precautions equipment: gloves, face shield, mask, etc.

One adult airway manikin for every five participants with the following:
—Lubricant for manikin (according to manufacturer)
—Adult bag-valve-mask system
—Mouth-to-mask device for ventilation
—End-tidal CO_2 detector (colormetric)
—Esophageal detection device
—Capnography equipment (optional)
—Pulse oximeter and probe (optional)
—Cardiac monitor/defibrillator/pacer system (optional)
—Oxygen supplement appliances: non-rebreather mask, simple mask, etc. (optional)
—Stethoscope
—Various adult-sized oropharyngeal airways
—Various adult-sized nasopharyngeal airways
—Dual-lumen combination tube (CombiTube) with syringes and gastric tube or PtL device with syringes
—Laryngeal mask airway (LMA), COBRA PLA or King LTD with appropriate syringes (optional)
—Adult-sized (various) endotracheal tubes with syringes and stylets
—Scenario medication kit with various sedative and paralytic agents (optional)

Instructor: Your role is important because you act as the coordinator of the station, assembling and troubleshooting equipment, and act as the facilitator of the scenario presented. Before the participant arrives, arrange equipment, lubricate manikin, check laryngoscope, etc. Please read the scenarios to become familiar with the necessary responses. As the scenario is introduced to the participants involved, answer questions asked but do not offer more information than would be obvious in looking at a patient.

Instructions

Hi, my name is _____, and I will be the instructor for this station. This is a hands-on patient assessment station. You will be given information concerning a patient experiencing a medical crisis. You will have all the necessary equipment you need to manage the patient in this station. Please look over the equipment before we go any further. You will be provided with pertinent information only when you ask the appropriate question. For any hands-on procedure, such as auscultation of a blood pressure or breath sounds or taking a pulse, select the appropriate equipment needed (if any) and use the equipment in the manner that it would be used on a patient. I will then give you the relevant clinical data. For example, you must select, place, and begin inflation of the BP cuff before the blood pressure is given to you. I will not answer questions in place of the patient. Therefore, it is imperative that you interact with your patient. Please verbalize to me any signs or symptoms that you find so that I will know you are cognizant of the patient and the patient's clinical appearance.

Scenario

Advise the participants that they are responding to a rural farm residence at 08:00 for an older gentleman whose wife states, "He won't wake up." If the participants are a nurses or in-hospital providers, this scenario can be modified to the medical environment—such as an elderly female drives up to the ED doors with her husband in the backseat of the car. The participants should use the assessment taught in this course.

Initial Impression: An elderly, thin male with his eyes closed; pale, no visible increased work of breathing.

Possible Differential (Field) Diagnoses: Altered mental status from stroke vs. shock vs. hypoxia vs. blood chemistry alteration vs. sepsis, etc.

Scene Size-up/General Impression: Century-old farmhouse with patient in upstairs bedroom. No scene hazards but potential for problems in getting this patient down the narrow steps. (Alternative: Patient in backseat of car—make sure car is off.) Frantic wife is present.

Initial Assessment:

Mental Status—Unresponsive to your verbal stimuli, extends to painful stimuli.

Airway—Some saliva in the mouth; intact gag reflex. Air is moving noisily.

Breathing—Slow rise and fall of the chest with shallow breath sounds only. Some loud, upper airway noise is heard.

Circulation—Radial pulses palpable at a slow rate.

Disability/Perfusion—Pupils are unequal: Right is at 6 mm, left is at 2 mm (no signs of cataracts). Extends to painful stimuli. Skin is cool and pale.

Status after Initial Assessment: Unstable, serious, potential life threat—needs immediate management.

Possible Differential (Field) Diagnoses: CNS event (elevated ICP, tumor, bleeding, stroke), CO toxicity, drug overdose, sepsis.

Initial Management Priorities: Immediate suctioning and assisted ventilations; after heart rate increases—cardiac monitor, IV therapy.

Focused History (SAMPLE):

Signs and Symptoms—Wife unable to awaken her husband. Felt OK yesterday.

Allergies—NKA.

Medications—Vitamins, otherwise no medications.

Previous History—"Broken leg when he was young"—otherwise no history. Hasn't seen a doctor in 20 years.

Last Oral Intake—Last night at about 6:00 P.M. (14 hours ago)

Events Preceding—Went to bed at usual time last evening. Nothing unusual.

OPQRST:

Onset—Sometime in the night.

Palliation/Provocation—Not applicable.

Quality—Not applicable.

Radiation—Not applicable.

Severity—Not applicable.

Time/Duration—Attempted to awaken him at 08:00—he usually rises at 06:00.

Vital Signs:
Respirations—6 breaths per minute, without assistance

Pulse—45 bpm prior to positive pressure ventilation (PPV) 80 bpm with PPV

Blood Pressure—180/110

Temperature—96°F (35.6°C)

Pulse Oximetry—85% on room air; 95% with PPV

Capnography—65 with spontaneous respirations; 40 with PPV

Blood Glucose Level—80 mg/dl (4.4 mmol/L)

Focused Physical Exam (Focused Medical Assessment): Rapid head-to-toe is negative except for unequal pupils, as described earlier. No signs of trauma.

Differential/Field Diagnosis: Hemorrhagic CVA

Management:
1) Immediate airway suctioning

2) Ventilatory assistance with high-flow oxygen at a rate of 12–15 per minute

3) IV access with minimal fluid administration

4) Cardiac and respiratory monitors

5) Advanced airway management with use of sedation vs. sedation and paralytic

6) Transport to the nearest appropriate medical center for stroke

Detailed Physical Exam: En route to appropriate facility as time permits.

Ongoing Assessment: There is no change in patient's condition during transport.

Critical Actions:
1) Basic and advanced airway techniques performed within the initial assessment for the basic techniques and the advanced techniques once the entire assessment and focused exam are completed.

2) Recognize the need for rapid transport of a critically ill patient with a time-critical medical problem.

Teaching Points

1) The assessment should point the participants towards a catastrophic, acute medical problem such as CVA. The instructor should review the differences in presentation of ischemic vs. hemorrhagic CVA. The instructor should also discuss differential diagnoses in the patient with acute loss of consciousness.

2) Because the patient postures with painful stimuli and has an intact gag reflex, providing an advanced airway may prove difficult. Use of RSI or alternative means of advanced airway management should be

discussed (e.g., nasotracheal route vs. RSI; use of sedation alone vs. use of sedation and paralytics). Discuss concerns regarding the increase in intracranial pressure.

3) Discussion should include whether to quickly facilitate transfer off the scene for a patient with a time-critical problem vs. staying and providing a more advanced airway, depending upon scene-hospital proximity.

Evaluation

1) *Excellent:* The participants were able to complete the medical assessment thoroughly, without prompting by the instructor. They were able to provide a field impression and differentials with tactics to rule in or out causes of unconsciousness. Critical thinking skills were attuned to providing basic and advanced airway management with thoughts towards scene time and proximity to an appropriate hospital and use of alternative advanced airway techniques vs. sedation only assistance vs. full RSI protocol use.

2) *Good:* The group was able to complete the medical assessment with minimal prompting by the instructor and with some organization. They were able to provide most of the differentials for the patient with acute unconsciousness and appropriate management for each. They were able to demonstrate good basic and advanced airway techniques. They were able to participate in the discussion, led by the instructor, on use of medication-assisted intubation, complications, and contraindications.

3) *Fair:* The participants were able to provide some aspects of the medical assessment and initial management without harm to the patient. Average knowledge in advanced airway techniques available to the patient in this case was demonstrated. Instructor had to lead most of the discussion on scene time for CVA vs. advanced airway management.

4) *Inadequate:* The group was unable to assess and manage the patient with acute unconsciousness, nor able to differentiate the possible causes. Their knowledge of management techniques for airway were lacking.

► Airway Management: Scenario 3

Requirements: One instructor and one manikin for every five participants.

Prerequisites: Read Chapter 2, "Airway Management, Ventilation, and Oxygen Therapy."

Airway (Optional) Scenarios: Equipment
Standard precautions equipment: gloves, face shield, mask, etc.

One adult airway manikin for every five participants with the following:
—Lubricant for manikin (according to manufacturer)
—Adult bag-valve-mask system
—Mouth-to-mask device for ventilation
—End-tidal CO_2 detector (colormetric)
—Esophageal detection device
—Capnography equipment (optional)
—Pulse oximeter and probe (optional)
—Cardiac monitor/defibrillator/pacer system (optional)
—Oxygen supplement appliances: non-rebreather mask, simple mask, etc.
  (optional)
—Stethoscope
—Various adult-sized oropharyngeal airways
—Various adult-sized nasopharyngeal airways
—Dual-lumen combination tube (CombiTube) with syringes and gastric
  tube or PtL device with syringes
—Laryngeal mask airway (LMA), COBRA PLA or King LTD with appro-
  priate syringes (optional)
—Adult-sized (various) endotracheal tubes with syringes and stylets
—Scenario medication kit with various sedative and paralytic agents (optional)

Instructor: Your role is important because you act as the coordinator of the station, assembling and troubleshooting equipment, and act as the facilitator of the scenario presented. Before the participant arrives, arrange equipment, lubricate manikin, check laryngoscope, etc. Please read the scenarios to become familiar with the necessary responses. As the scenario is introduced to the participants involved, answer questions asked but do not offer more information than would be obvious in looking at a patient.

Instructions

Hi, my name is _____, and I will be the instructor for this station. This is a hands-on patient assessment station. You will be given information concerning a patient experiencing a medical crisis. You will have all the necessary equipment you need to manage the patient in this station. Please look over the equipment before we go any further. You will be provided with pertinent information only when you ask the appropriate question. For any hands-on procedure, such as auscultation of a blood pressure or breath sounds or taking a pulse, select the appropriate equipment needed (if any) and use the equipment in the manner that it would be used on a patient. I will then give you the relevant clinical data. For example, you must select, place, and begin inflation of the BP cuff before the blood pressure is given to you. I will not answer questions in place of the patient. Therefore, it is imperative that you interact with your patient. Please verbalize to me any signs or symptoms that you find so that I will know you are cognizant of the patient and the patient's clinical appearance.

Scenario

The participants are responding to a 911 request for "a lady who is swelling up." Upon arrival at a local shopping area, you find a 55-year-old very anxious female standing near the front entrance of a small restaurant. The scene appears safe.

If the participants are in-hospital care workers, this could be the same female who has arrived at the registration/triage area of your emergency department.

Initial Impression: Anxious female in obvious respiratory distress with noticeable facial and lip swelling—tongue is distended and there is drooling.

Possible Differential (Field) Diagnoses: Anaphylaxis vs. allergic reaction vs. angioedema vs. trauma.

Scene Size-up/General Impression: Critical situation in a safe scene.

Initial Assessment:

Mental Status—Responsive and anxious. Standing up—won't sit down.

Airway—Some air moving but with increased work of breathing. Drooling.

Breathing—Rapid and labored breathing—shallow breath sounds.

Circulation—Radial pulses palpable in periphery—fast.

Disability/Perfusion—Patient unable to speak but nods head appropriately to questions. Follows commands. Skin warm and dry.

Status after Initial Assessment: Unstable, serious, potential life threat—needs immediate management.

Possible Differential (Field) Diagnoses: Angioedema (acute allergic reaction, hereditary, drug-induced), oral infection (including epiglottitis), trauma, insect sting/bite.

Initial Management Priorities: Cautious airway management with supplemental oxygen.

Focused History (SAMPLE):

Signs and Symptoms—Bystander reports fairly rapid onset of swelling that began while eating.

Allergies—Shrimp, bananas, and many other environmental allergies.

Medications—ACE inhibitor.

Previous History—Hypertension.

Last Oral Intake—Eating at onset of symptoms.

Events Preceding—Eating, then complained of some nausea with "hot" feeling in her face.

OPQRST:

Onset—20 minutes ago

Palliation/Provocation—Sitting down makes it worse

Quality—Not applicable—no pain

Radiation—Not applicable

Severity—Not applicable

Time/Duration—20 minutes of steadily increasing airway compromise

Vital Signs:

   Respirations—30, shallow and labored

   Pulse—120 per minute

   Blood Pressure—160/110

   Temperature—98.6°F (37°C)

   Pulse Oximetry—90% on room air, 94% with supplemental oxygen

   Capnography—45 mmHg

   Blood Glucose Level—100 mg/dl (5.5 mmol/L)

Focused Physical Exam (Focused Medical Assessment): Rapid head-to-toe is negative except for facial, lip edema with erythema and swollen tongue with drooling. No signs of trauma.

Differential/Field Diagnosis: Allergic reaction—probable angioedema

Management:

1) Immediate (cautious) airway suctioning—possibly patient controlled. Position of preference to maintain best respiratory status.

2) High-flow oxygen at a rate of 12–15 per minute as tolerated with positive pressure ventilation immediately available should level of consciousness deteriorate.

3) IV access with minimal fluid administration (unless blood pressure drops).

4) Use of the Allergic Reaction protocol with possible use of Epineph-rine, Diphenhydramine and/or steroids, as directed. Beta-2 Agonists if wheezing.

5) Cardiac and respiratory monitors

6) Prepare for advanced airway management. Rapid sequence induction (RSI)/sedation is contra-indicated.

7) Transport to the nearest appropriate medical center for advanced air-way management.

Detailed Physical Exam: En route to appropriate facility as time permits.

Ongoing Assessment: There is no change in patient's condition during transport.

Critical Actions:

1) Basic airway techniques performed within the initial assessment. Transport should begin quickly thereafter. The provider should be quite cautious about attempting advanced or even basic airway management with adjuncts with this patient.

2) Recognize the need for rapid transport of a critically ill patient with a time-critical medical problem and the provider's understanding of the need for caution.

Teaching Points

1) The assessment should point the participants towards a potentially catastrophic, acute medical problem such as angioedema. The instructor should review the pathophysiology of angioedema, food allergies, and the incidence of ACE inhibitor use and angioedema. The instructor

should also discuss differential diagnoses in the patient with this type of quick-onset, edematous airway and use of allergic reaction protocols: Epinephrine and Diphenhydramine or steroid use, Beta-2 agonist if reactive airway signs are present.

2) Because the patient postures herself in a standing position the provider should also be rational in patient positioning for transport. Advanced airway may prove quite difficult even for the most experienced anesthesiologists. Use of RSI or alternative means of advanced airway management should be discussed (e.g., high-risk prehospital RSI vs. judicious transport to advanced airway resources in a controlled setting), but the advanced-level participants should recognize a patient who should not have RSI done in the field. The instructor should ask the providers what they would do, should the patient's condition deteriorate. Bag-mask ventilation should be encouraged.

3) Discussion should include whether to quickly facilitate transfer off the scene for a patient with a time-critical problem vs. staying and delaying a more advanced airway, depending upon scene-hospital proximity.

Evaluation

1) *Excellent:* The participants were able to complete the medical assessment thoroughly, without prompting by the instructor. They were able to provide a field impression and differentials with tactics to rule in or out causes of rapid airway compromise. Critical thinking skills were attuned to providing basic airway management with thoughts towards scene time and transport to an appropriate hospital and possible use of the Allergic Reaction protocols. Able to discuss within the group, preparations in the event of patient deterioration.

2) *Good:* The group was able to complete the medical assessment with minimal prompting by the instructor and with some organization. They were able to provide most of the differentials for the patient with acute airway edema and appropriate management for each. They were able to demonstrate good basic airway techniques. They were able to participate in the discussion, led by the instructor, on being prepared for actions should the patient's condition deteriorate.

3) *Fair:* The participants were able to provide some aspects of the medical assessment and initial management without harm to the patient. Average knowledge in airway techniques available to the patient in this case was demonstrated. Instructor had to lead most of the discussion on angioedema, cautious airway management, and the recognition of a patient that should be transported without an advanced airway.

4) *Inadequate:* The group was unable to assess and manage the patient with acute airway compromise, nor able to differentiate the possible causes. Their knowledge of management techniques for airway were lacking or too aggressive and cavalier for the situation.

► AIRWAY MANAGEMENT: SCENARIO 4

Requirements: One instructor and one manikin for every five participants.

Prerequisites: Read Chapter 2, "Airway Management, Ventilation, and Oxygen Therapy."

Airway (Optional) Scenarios: Equipment
Standard precautions equipment: gloves, face shield, mask, etc.

One adult airway manikin for every 5 participants with the following:
—Lubricant for manikin (according to manufacturer)
—Adult bag-valve-mask system
—Mouth-to-mask device for ventilation
—End-tidal CO_2 detector (colormetric)
—Esophageal detection device
—Capnography equipment (optional)
—Pulse oximeter and probe (optional)
—Cardiac monitor/defibrillator/pacer system (optional)
—Oxygen supplement appliances: non-rebreather mask, simple mask, etc. (optional)
—Stethoscope
—Various adult-sized oropharyngeal airways
—Various adult-sized nasopharyngeal airways
—Dual-lumen combination tube (CombiTube) with syringes and gastric tube or PtL device with syringes
—Laryngeal mask airway (LMA), COBRA PLA or King LTD with appropriate syringes (optional)
—Adult-sized (various) endotracheal tubes with syringes and stylets
—Scenario medication kit with various sedative and paralytic agents (optional)

Instructor: Your role is important because you act as the coordinator of the station, assembling and troubleshooting equipment, and act as the facilitator of the scenario presented. Before the participant arrives, arrange equipment, lubricate manikin, check laryngoscope, etc. Please read the scenarios to become familiar with the necessary responses. As the scenario is introduced to the participants involved, answer questions asked but do not offer more information than would be obvious in looking at a patient.

Instructions

Hi, my name is _____, and I will be the instructor for this station. This is a hands-on patient assessment station. You will be given information concerning a patient experiencing a medical crisis. You will have all the necessary equipment you need to manage the patient in this station. Please look over the equipment before we go any further. You will be provided with pertinent information only when you ask the appropriate question. For any hands-on procedure, such as auscultation of a blood pressure or breath sounds or taking a pulse, select the appropriate equipment needed (if any) and use the equipment in the manner that it would be used on a patient. I will then give you the relevant clinical data. For example, you must select, place, and begin inflation of the BP cuff before the blood pressure is given to you. I will not answer questions in place of the patient. Therefore, it is imperative that you interact with your patient. Please verbalize to me any signs or symptoms that you find so that I will know you are cognizant of the patient and the patient's clinical appearance.

Scenario

You are responding to a report of a patient breathing "funny." Dispatch informs you that they are now giving pre-arrival instructions to the family of this patient with emphasis on airway management.

If the participants are in-hospital providers, the instructor may revise the scenario to allow for the arrival of a large utility vehicle with a sick patient in the rear compartment, driving up to the triage door.

Initial Impression: A middle-aged male patient is found on a bed in the living room (or the rear area of a utility vehicle). He appears Pickwickian (severely obese) and in severe respiratory distress. Family is in attendance report that he is approximately 5 feet tall (152 cm) and 800 pounds (360 Kg).

Possible Differential (Field) Diagnoses: Positional airway compromise with respiratory failure; respiratory compromise due to infection, infarction, aspiration, allergy, etc.

Scene Size-up/General Impression: Critical. Safe scene but special resources necessary for moving this patient. Participants should ask for additional help early.

Initial Assessment:

Mental Status—Eyes closed, flutters eyelids to painful stimuli.

Airway—Snoring sound with large amount of soft tissue vibration in face and neck.

Breathing—Rapid and labored breathing—shallow breath sounds.

Circulation—Difficult to find due to tissue layers.

Disability/Perfusion—GCS 3. No spontaneous movement, other than breathing. Skin cool and dry.

Status after Initial Assessment: Unstable, serious, potential life threat—needs immediate management.

Possible Differential (Field) Diagnoses: Exacerbation of COPD, pneumonia, pulmonary embolism, CHF, MI, upper airway obstruction (including obstructive sleep apnea), aspiration, CNS event (e.g., stroke), drug overdose, hypoglycemia.

Initial Management Priorities: Immediate airway and ventilatory management with special resources. Bag and mask ventilation should be instituted immediately with supplemental oxygen applied when available. Two- to three-person bag and mask technique recommended.

Focused History (SAMPLE):

Signs and Symptoms—Family reports that the patient's Continuous Positive Airway Pressure (CPAP) machine "quit working" 2 days ago and they found him "like this" 30 minutes ago when they went to rouse him.

Allergies—No known allergies.

Medications—Beta-1 blocker and calcium-channel blocker for hypertension, and "stomach medicine" for heartburn.

Previous History—Hypertension and stomach problems, obesity with sleep apnea.

Last Oral Intake—02:00, he ate a chicken meal.

Events Preceding—Went to bed (special bed in the living room) at about 03:00 and wouldn't wake up at 08:00 A.M.

OPQRST:

Onset—20 minutes ago, wouldn't awaken

Palliation/Provocation—Not applicable

Quality—Not applicable—no complaint of pain

Radiation—Not applicable

Severity—Not applicable

Time/Duration—Found 20 minutes ago

Vital Signs:

Respirations—20, labored with very little air movement heard

Pulse—60 and difficult to palpate

Blood Pressure—no cuff to fit patient's arm—large arm cuff on forearm shows: 100/40

Temperature—96.2°F (35.7°C)

Pulse Oximetry—Poor pleth; occasionally reads 88% with patient receiving supplemental oxygen

Capnography—80

Blood Glucose Level—200 mg/dl (11 mmol/L)

Focused Physical Exam (Focused Medical Assessment): Rapid head-to-toe reveals no signs of trauma. Obese male with positional airway obstruction.

Differential/Field Diagnosis: Presumed respiratory failure from airway obstruction; possible stroke, vs. metabolic derangement

Management:

1) Immediate head-tilt, chin lift with bag and mask ventilation. Two-person bag and mask with one person providing cricoid pressure. Supplemental oxygen applied when available.

2) Airway adjunct—the participants may try any technique that they think will work here AND is within their scope of practice. Those wishing to intubate should describe the special techniques they will use to successfully view this patient's cords, given the redundant soft tissue problems. Options that might work include basic airways with bag and mask, supraglottic airways (LMA, King LTD, Cobra, etc.), digital intubation, or transporting patient with simplest airway that works.

3) IV access with minimal fluid administration.

4) Cardiac and respiratory monitors.

5) Rule out reversible conditions: hypoglycemia, opioid toxicity.

Detailed Physical Exam: En route to appropriate facility as time and space permit.

Ongoing Assessment: There is no change in patient's condition during transport as long as appropriate airway and ventilatory management are being provided.

Critical Actions:

1) Basic airway techniques performed within the initial assessment. Transport should begin as soon as resources available to safely move this large patient. The provider should be able to discuss and plan for airway, ventilation, and transportation issues.

2) Safe and efficient movement of a very large patient while providing resuscitation. This requires pre-planning and logistical tactics with tact.

Teaching Points

1) This is a patient who will expire quickly if the group does not provide basic airway and ventilatory support. Discussion about the airway challenge present in these types of patients is the main goal of this scenario and the instructor must allow for discussion and possibly hands-on demonstration of alternative airway techniques. The airway discourse should include "ramping up" procedures (propping the large patient into a 30–40° head-up position from waist to crown) in order to reduce the redundant tissue of the face and throat. It should also include use of larger intubation equipment, alternative techniques and devices (as already listed), and use of CPAP in the pre-hospital setting.

2) The instructor discusses Pickwick Syndrome and sleep apnea, and home use of CPAP and BiPAP for these patients.

3) Tactful and professional management of this situation should also be emphasized. The overall coordination and logistical maneuvering that needs to occur while moving a patient of this size can be overwhelming without some pre-planning. The instructor might want to emphasize some pre-planning ideas with the group or call upon members of the group that have completed these special transfers. Many times, they are completed as part of a "routine" transfer, but in this case, a true emergency exists and time on the scene should be considered along with safety.

Evaluation

1) *Excellent:* The participants evaluated and recognized the need for a secure airway and ventilation prior to arranging for transport. They worked as a team to complete the medical assessment of the patient including SAMPLE, OPQRST, and a focused exam. They assessed for the cause of the patient's altered mental status, using the AMLS techniques taught. They demonstrated good skills and discussed appropriate monitoring and ventilation technique. Their discussion about the logistics of transporting large patients was constructive and professional.

2) *Good:* The group evaluated the patient using the standard medical assessment format and recognized the patient with a decreased level of consciousness with airway compromise and respiratory failure. They displayed an above-average knowledge of airway management and alternatives for this patient's condition. They were able to perform the skills of airway and ventilation management and discussed with the instructor the steps necessary to transport a large patient.

3) *Fair:* The group evaluated the patient with some assistance from the instructor. They recognized the need for airway and ventilation management but had to be coached on how to perform these procedures. They followed the lead of the instructor in assessing for the special challenges of this airway management. They could provide basic airway and ventilation skills with assistance and had to be taught the pathophysiology of the case.

4) *Inadequate:* The entire station had to be taught by the instructor. The group was unable to provide a medical assessment, unable to identify pathophysiology, and unable to appropriately manage the basics without being led by the instructor.

⊞ HYPOPERFUSION (SHOCK)

▶ HYPOPERFUSION (SHOCK): SCENARIO 1

Requirements: One instructor and one patient for every five participants.

Prerequisites: Read Chapter 4, "Hypoperfusion (Shock)."

Equipment: One table and chair for the patient to use; jump kit with oxygen supplies (NC, NRM, aerosol mask, PPV device, intubation equipment), stethoscope, BP cuff, cardiac monitor, pulse oximeter, and medication kit with assorted medications.

Instructor: Your role is vital because you must act as the coordinator of the station and also interact in the scenario. Before the participant arrives at the station, please review the scenario with your patient. Spray the patient's arms with a fine mist of cool water to simulate cool and clammy skin.

Patient: One male (or female) patient. As the patient, you will be required to play the role of a 46-year-old male suffering from difficulty breathing. You will be awake and alert and answer all questions. Please read the scenario to familiarize yourself with the information. You will have a fine mist of water sprayed on you to simulate cool and diaphoretic skin. Moulage is used to simulate pale skin.

Instructions

Hi, my name is _____, and I will be the instructor for this station. This is a hands-on patient assessment station. You will be given information concerning a patient experiencing a medical crisis. You will have all the necessary equipment you need to manage the patient in this station. Please look over the equipment before we go any further. You will be provided with pertinent information only when you ask the appropriate question. For any hands-on procedure, such as auscultation of a blood pressure or breath sounds or taking a pulse, select the appropriate equipment needed (if any) and use the equipment in the manner that it would be used on a patient. I will then give you the relevant clinical data. For example, you must select, place, and begin inflation of the BP cuff before the blood pressure is given to you. I will not answer questions in place of the patient. Therefore, it is imperative that you interact with your patient. Please verbalize to me any signs or symptoms that you find so that I will know you are cognizant of the patient and the patient's clinical appearance.

Scenario

Advise the participants that they are responding to a call of an unknown medical emergency in residential neighborhood at the beginning of their shift. If the participants are nurses or in-hospital providers, the scenario can be modified to the medical environment—such as reporting to triage after shift change and being told that a patient with abdominal pain has just walked into Medical Room 5. The participant should use the assessment taught in this course.

Initial Impression: 46-year-old male (or female) sitting up in bed at residence.

Scene Size-up/General Impression: Patient appears frightened and having difficulty breathing. Potentially unstable patient, no apparent injury noted; there are no scene safety issues present.

Initial Assessment:

Mental Status—A&O × 3, answering questions appropriately.

Airway—Clear and patent at this time.

Breathing—Respirations labored, rapid, and shallow with crackles in all four lobes. Patient denies a productive cough.

Circulation—Radial pulse is regular and slow.

Disability/Perfusion—Moves all four extremities. Skin warm, dry, and pink.

Status after Initial Assessment: Stable, potential for deteriorating and becoming a life threat.

Possible Differential (Field) Diagnoses: cardiovascular emergency/CHF, pulmonary edema, COPD, pneumonia, bronchitis, anaphylaxis, and ARDS toxicology emergencies. Encourage participants to share other possible etiologies.

Initial Management Priorities: High-flow oxygen at 15 lpm via NRM, cardiac monitor, IV access, position of comfort.

Focused History (SAMPLE):

Signs and Symptoms—Difficulty in breathing. Patient more comfortable in high-fowler's position. Patient denies chest pain and any numbness or tingling in extremities.

Allergies—Penicillin.

Medications—Patient is prescribed propranolol (Inderal) 80 mg extended-release PO daily, but has been taking three times the daily dose (240 mg) over several days. Patient admits to not understanding dosage instructions. Patient was prescribed medication 3 days ago.

Past Medical History—Hypertension, angina pectoris. AMI 2 years ago.

Last Oral Intake—Patient had a light dinner last evening.

Events Preceding—Patient hasn't felt well for a couple of days. He woke this morning with difficulty breathing.

OPQRST:

Onset—Gradual, over a couple of days.

Palliation/Provocation—I feel better sitting upright and not moving.

Quality—Breathing discomfort worsens with exertion and laying flat.

Radiation—Discomfort is localized to entire chest.

Severity—Patient identifies as a 7 on a 0–10 scale.

Time/Duration—Breathing difficulty started about 48 hours ago.

Vital Signs:

Respirations—12 and labored, crackles in all four lobes

Pulse—Radial pulse weak at 48 bpm

Blood Pressure—68/52

Temperature—98.4°F (36.9°C)

Pulse Oximetry—90

Blood Glucose Level—72 mg/dl (4.0 mmol/L)

Focused Physical Exam (Focused Medical Assessment): Minimal pedal edema, weak distal pulses, motor and sensory exam unremarkable.

Differential/Field Diagnosis: Cardiogenic shock related to slow rate and decreased myocardial contractility in response to the direct effect of beta 1 blockade on heart, resulting in hypoperfusion.

Management:
1) High-flow oxygen at 15 lpm via NRM.

2) IV therapy at TKO rate with constant evaluation of lung sounds. If lungs are clear and patient is hypotensive, give IV fluids cautiously.

3) Cardiac monitor—sinus bradycardia with no ectopy.

4) External (or transvenous pacing) for severe cases.

5) Atropine.

6) Glucagon.

7) Activated charcoal, especially if recent ingestion.

8) Consider calcium IV.

9) Dopamine 5–15 µg/kg/min titrated to keep systolic between 70–100 mmHg or other catecholamine if in hospital.

10) Rapid transport to appropriate facility (may need aortic balloon, transvenous pacing).

Detailed Physical Exam: En route to appropriate facility if time permits.

Ongoing Assessment: There is no change in patient's condition during transport.

Critical Actions:
1) Secure the airway and ensure oxygenation at 15 lpm via NRM; if respiratory failure, then PPV.

2) Maintain hemodynamic stability—BP between 70–100 mmHg, no higher.

3) Cardiac pacing if hypoperfusion severe.

Teaching Points

1) Hypoperfusion from cardiogenic shock due to excessive beta blocker intake. Beta 1 receptor block in the heart decreases rate and contractility.

2) Some beta blockers such as propranolol pass through blood brain barrier and into the CNS, leading to decreased mental status and seizures, and may lead to respiratory depression.

3) Elderly and immunocompromised patients are at risk for hypothermia.

4) Other drugs that lead to cardiogenic shock and cause CNS dysfunction are: exposure to agricultural insecticides (carbonates), heroin, and toxic levels of prescribed drugs.

5) Cardiac dysrhythmias should be managed according to current American Heart Association (AHA) ACLS guidelines.

6) Propranolol can mask many of the typical signs and symptoms of shock and hypoglycemia, such as tremor, tachycardia, and agitation.

7) Always follow an organized approach to rule out possible causes.

Evaluation

1) *Excellent:* The participant's evaluation of the patient followed set format: initial assessment, focused history (SAMPLE, OPQRST) in an efficient manner. The participant displayed a thorough knowledge of the patient's condition, performed the exam and management in an organized manner, and demonstrated an excellent overall performance.

2) *Good:* The participant's evaluation of the patient followed set format: initial assessment, focused history (SAMPLE, OPQRST) in an acceptable manner with only minor deviation. The participant displayed an above-average knowledge of the patient's condition, performed the exam and management of the patient's condition, and demonstrated an above-average performance.

3) *Fair:* The participant's evaluation of the patient deviated from the set format without causing any further injury to the patient. The participant displayed an average or basic knowledge of the patient's condition and performed an adequate exam and management of the patient's condition.

4) *Inadequate:* The participant's evaluation of the patient deviated significantly from the set format, or the participant's actions endangered the patient's life or significantly exacerbated the condition.

▶ Hypoperfusion (Shock): Scenario 2

Requirements: One instructor and one patient for every five participants.

Prerequisites: Read Chapter 4, "Hypoperfusion (Shock)."

Equipment: One table and chair for the patient to use; jump kit with oxygen supplies (NC, NRM, aerosol mask, PPV device, intubation equipment), stethoscope, BP cuff, cardiac monitor, pulse oximeter, and medication kit with assorted medications.

Instructor: Your role is vital because you must act as the coordinator of the station and also interact in the scenario. Before the participant arrives at the station, please review the scenario with your patient. Spray the patient's arms with a fine mist of cool water to simulate cool and clammy skin.

Patient: One female patient. As the patient, you will be required to play the role of a 26-year-old female complaining of difficulty breathing. You will be responsive and answer all questions. Please read the scenario to familiarize yourself with all the information. You will have a fine mist of water sprayed on you to simulate cool and diaphoretic skin.

Instructions

Hi, my name is _____, and I will be the instructor for this station. This is a hands-on patient assessment station. You will be given information concerning a patient experiencing a medical crisis. You will have all the necessary equipment you need to manage the patient in this station. Please look over the equipment before we go any further. You will be provided with pertinent information only when you ask the appropriate question. For any hands-on procedure, such as auscultation of a blood pressure or breath sounds or taking a pulse, select the appropriate equipment needed (if any) and use the equipment in the manner that it would be used on a patient. I will then give you the relevant clinical data. For example, you must select, place, and begin inflation of the BP cuff before the blood pressure is given to you. I will not answer questions in place of the patient. Therefore, it is imperative that you interact with your patient. Please verbalize to me any signs or symptoms that you find so that I will know you are cognizant of the patient and the patient's clinical appearance.

Scenario

Advise the participants that they are responding to a call for difficulty breathing at a local bus depot. If the participants are nurses or in-hospital providers, the scenario can be modified to the medical environment—such as having a taxi driver pull up to the ED doors and ask for assistance in removing the patient. The participants should use the assessment taught in the course.

Initial Impression: 26-year-old female, awake and alert and able to answer questions.

Scene Size-up/General Impression: Ill female sitting on the curb next to the bus. No evidence of trauma.

Initial Assessment:
  Mental Status—Responsive and alert to all commands. Patient is anxious, restless, and agitated.

  Airway—Clear and patent at this time.

Breathing—Respirations 46 and very shallow.

Circulation—Radial pulse irregular at 106 bpm.

Disability/Perfusion—Moves all four extremities. Skin is cool and diaphoretic.

Status after Initial Assessment: Unstable, potential life threat.

Possible Differential (Field) Diagnoses: Respiratory compromise from anaphylaxis, respiratory infection, pulmonary embolus, pneumothorax, pneumonia, pulmonary edema (cardiac or non-cardiac), cardiovascular emergency, psychogenic disturbance. Encourage participants to offer additional possibilities for etiologies.

Initial Management Priorities: High-flow oxygen at 15 lpm via NRM, percuss lung sounds, cardiac monitor, IV access, position of comfort.

Focused History (SAMPLE):

Signs and Symptoms—Patient sitting upright and leaning forward, shallow respirations, cool and clammy skin.

Allergies—Aspirin.

Medications—Birth control.

Past Medical History—Patient has smoked two packs of cigarettes a day for 10 years.

Last Oral Intake—A hamburger and fries at bus stop diner about 2 hours ago.

Events Preceding—Patient stated she developed a sharp pain in her chest after she stood up and got off the bus. (If the participant inquires further, the bus trip was 16 hours long.)

OPQRST:

Onset—Very sudden, when I stood up.

Palliation/Provocation—Anytime I move from a sitting position, it gets worse. Deep inspiration increases pain.

Quality—It's very sharp.

Radiation—It's just in my chest.

Severity—The pain and difficulty breathing rank a 7 on a 0–10 scale.

Time—It's been going on for about 20 minutes.

Vital Signs:

Respirations—46 and shallow

Pulse—Radial pulse irregular at 102 bpm

Blood Pressure—84/76

Temperature—98.5°F (37.0°C)

Pulse Oximetry—91%

Focused Physical Exam (Focused Medical Assessment): Unremarkable. Diminished lungs sounds. Distal pulses weak and irregular.

Differential/Field Diagnosis: Obstructive shock (pulmonary embolism)

Management:

1) High-flow oxygen at 15 lpm via NRM

2) IV access—fluid bolus to maintain a systolic BP of 70–100 mmHg

3) Cardiac monitor—sinus tachycardia with multifocal PVCs

4) Transport in position of comfort.

5) Vasopressors (e.g., dopamine) if necessary

6) Rapid testing for PE—consider empiric anti-coagulation

Detailed Physical Exam: En route to appropriate facility if time permits.

Ongoing Assessment: Continue to monitor respiratory status. Monitor vital signs.

Critical Actions:

1) Secure the airway and ensure highest oxygenation at 15 lpm via NRM; if respiratory failure, then PPV.

2) Maintain hemodynamic stability—BP between 70–100 mmHg, no higher.

Teaching Points

1) History of oral birth control, heavy smoker, and being sedentary puts patient at risk for pulmonary embolus (also obesity, history of deep vein thrombosis [DVT], long travel).

2) Pulmonary emboli often have chest pain that is pleuritic in nature.

3) Tachycardia results from compensation for decreased preload, tachypnea results from compensation from hypoxia. A normal pulse oximetry reading does not rule out pulmonary embolus diagnosis.

4) Always follow an organized approach to rule out possible causes.

Evaluation

1) *Excellent:* The participant's evaluation of the patient followed set format: initial assessment, focused history (SAMPLE, OPQRST) in an efficient manner. The participant displayed a thorough knowledge of the patient's condition, performed the exam and management in an organized manner, and demonstrated an excellent overall performance.

2) *Good:* The participant's evaluation of the patient followed set format: initial assessment, focused history (SAMPLE, OPQRST) in an acceptable manner with only minor deviation. The participant displayed an above-average knowledge of the patient's condition, performed the exam and management of the patient's condition, and demonstrated an above-average performance.

3) *Fair:* The participant's evaluation of the patient deviated from the set format without causing any further injury to the patient. The participant displayed an average or basic knowledge of the patient's condition and performed an adequate exam and management of the patient's condition.

4) *Inadequate:* The participant's evaluation of the patient deviated significantly from the set format, or the participant's actions endangered the patient's life or significantly exacerbated the condition.

▶ HYPOPERFUSION (SHOCK): SCENARIO 3

Requirements: One instructor and one patient for every five participants.

Prerequisites: Read Chapter 4, "Hypoperfusion (Shock)."

Equipment: One table and chair for the patient to use; jump kit with oxygen supplies (NC, NRM, aerosol mask, PPV device, intubation equipment), stethoscope, BP cuff, cardiac monitor, pulse oximeter, and medication kit with assorted medications

Instructor: Your role is vital because you must act as the coordinator of the station and also interact in the scenario. You will also act as the nurse who is responsible for this patient. When EMS arrives, you state that the patient has had a high fever (104.2°F/40.4°C) for approximately 12 hours that has not been relieved with Tylenol. The doctor was notified because the patient was no longer responsive, and ordered the patient sent to the ED for evaluation. After that you can tell the participant that you must tend to another patient and will no longer be available. Before the participants arrive at the station, please review the scenario with your patient.

Patient: One female (or male) patient. As the patient, you will be required to play the role of a 74-year-old female suffering from an elevated temperature. You will be responsive only to painful stimuli with purposeful movement (attempt to move away from the pain). Please read the scenario to familiarize yourself with the information.

Instructions

Hi, my name is _____, and I will be the instructor for this station. This is a hands-on patient assessment station. You will be given information concerning a patient experiencing a medical crisis. You will have all the necessary equipment you need to manage the patient in this station. Please look over the equipment before we go any further. You will be provided with pertinent information only when you ask the appropriate question. For any hands-on procedure, such as auscultation of a blood pressure or breath sounds or taking a pulse, select the appropriate equipment needed (if any) and use the equipment in the manner that it would be used on a patient. I will then give you the relevant clinical data. For example, you must select, place, and begin inflation of the BP cuff before the blood pressure is given to you. I will not answer questions in place of the patient. Therefore, it is imperative that you interact with your patient. Please verbalize to me any signs or symptoms that you find so that I will know you are cognizant of the patient and the patient's clinical appearance.

Scenario

Advise the participants that they are responding to a call at the local nursing home for a "resident who is ill." If the participants are nurses or in-hospital providers, the scenario can be modified to the medical environment—such as reporting to triage after a shift change where the patient is found near the triage desk slumped over in a wheelchair. The participant should use the assessment taught in this course.

Initial Impression: 82-year-old female (or male) nursing home patient lying in bed.

Scene Size-up/General Impression: There are no apparent signs of injury on brief visual exam. Wheelchairs have been moved for easy access to patient.

Initial Assessment:

    Mental Status—Purposeful attempt to remove painful stimulus.

    Airway—Clear at this time.

    Breathing—Respirations rapid and very shallow, crackles in the bases.

    Circulation—Radial pulse is weak and thready, barely palpable.

    Disability/Perfusion—Withdrawal from pain in all four extremities. Skin is warm and dry to the touch.

Status after Initial Assessment: Unstable, potential life threat.

Possible Differential (Field) Diagnoses: Altered mental status from sepsis, pneumonia, toxicological emergency, hypo/hyperglycemia, environmental emergencies, CNS compromise, CHF. Encourage participants to share other possible etiologies.

Initial Management Priorities: High-flow oxygen at 15 lpm via NRM, IV access, cardiac monitor, position of comfort.

Focused History (SAMPLE):

    Signs and Symptoms—Responsive only to painful stimuli, weak radial pulse, warm and dry skin, crackles in the bases of the lungs

    Allergies—On transfer sheet, penicillin, amoxicillin, vancomycin

    Medications—On transfer sheet, Humulin N, aspirin, Cardizem

    Past Medical History—On transfer sheet, Insulin Dependent Diabetes Meuitus (IDDM), and atrial fibrillation

    Last Oral Intake—Unknown

    Events Preceding—Already stated by nurse who left the room

OPQRST:

    Onset—About 12 hours ago

    Palliation/Provocation—Unknown

    Quality—Unknown

    Radiation—Unknown

    Severity—Unknown

    Time—Unknown

Vital Signs:

    Respirations—36 and very shallow

    Pulse—Radial pulse rapid and weak at 116 bpm

    Blood Pressure—68/palpation

    Temperature—104.6°F (40.7°C)

    Pulse Oximetry—Reading error

    Blood Glucose Level—86 mg/dl (4.7 mmol/L)

Focused Physical Exam (Focused Medical Assessment): No injury. Bruising from insulin injections noted on left upper quadrant of abdomen. Large decubitus ulcer on right thigh and buttocks.

Differential/Field Diagnosis: Distributive shock (sepsis)

Management:

1) Supplemental oxygen at 15 lpm via NRM; if respiratory failure, then PPV

2) IV access, fluid boluses to maintain a systolic BP between 70–100 mmHg

3) Cardiac monitor—atrial fibrillation

4) Consider dopamine 5–10 µg/kg/min to increase pressure

5) Transport

Detailed Physical Exam: Rapid head-to-toe physical exam to identify potential for abuse, neglect, or previous injury

Ongoing Assessment: There is no change in patient's condition during transport.

Critical Actions:

1) Secure airway and ensure oxygenation at 15 lpm via NRM; if respiratory failure, then PPV.

2) Maintain hemodynamic stability—BP between 70–100 mmHg.

Teaching Points

1) There are numerous causes and etiologies of hypoperfusion/shock.

2) Elderly are at risk for sepsis due to their inability to compensate, body's defense mechanisms are easily overwhelmed, and many chronic illnesses, such as diabetes mellitus.

3) Septic shock signs and symptoms can be subtle. Elderly may not exhibit a fever. Skin can be flushed and pink (due to fever) or pale and cyanotic in later stages of septic shock. Petechiae rash can often be evident from development of microemboli. Alteration in mental status is often an early sign.

4) Increased permeability and vasodilation can alter lung sounds and be confused with the signs and symptoms of congested heart failure.

5) Always follow an organized approach to rule out possible causes.

6) Treatment priorities are to maintain oxygenation and hemodynamic stability.

Evaluation

1) *Excellent:* The participant's evaluation of the patient followed set format: initial assessment, focused history (SAMPLE, OPQRST) in an efficient manner. The participant displayed a thorough knowledge of the patient's condition, performed the exam and management in an organized manner, and demonstrated an excellent overall performance.

2) *Good:* The participant's evaluation of the patient followed set format: initial assessment, focused history (SAMPLE, OPQRST) in an acceptable manner with only minor deviation. The participant displayed an above-average knowledge of the patient's condition, performed the exam and management of the patient's condition, and demonstrated an above-average performance.

3) *Fair:* The participant's evaluation of the patient deviated from the set format without causing any further injury to the patient. The participant displayed an average or basic knowledge of the patient's condition and performed an adequate exam and management of the patient's condition.

4) *Inadequate:* The participant's evaluation of the patient deviated significantly from the set format, or the participant's actions endangered the patient's life or significantly exacerbated the condition.

▶ Hypoperfusion (Shock): Scenario 4

Requirements: One instructor and one patient for every five participants

Prerequisites: Read Chapter 4, "Hypoperfusion (Shock)."

Equipment: One table and chair for the patient to use; jump kit with oxygen supplies (NC, NRM, aerosol mask, PPV device, intubation equipment), stethoscope, BP cuff, cardiac monitor, pulse oximeter, and medication kit with assorted medications.

Instructor: Your role is vital because you must act as the coordinator of the station and also interact in the scenario. Before the participant arrives at the station, please review the scenario with your patient. For moulage, tint the patient's arms and anterior chest red to simulate erythema.

Patient: One male (or female) patient. As the patient, you will be required to play the role of a 28-year-old male suffering from difficulty in breathing and increasing signs of shock due to an anaphylactic reaction from a bee sting. You are alert and very agitated. When asked questions, you are initially able to communicate but with great difficulty. You were cutting grass when you felt a burning in your leg. Please read the scenario to familiarize yourself with the information.

Instructions

Hi, my name is _____, and I will be the instructor this station. This is a hands-on patient assessment station. You will be given information concerning a patient experiencing a medical crisis. You will have all the necessary equipment you need to manage the patient in this station. Please look over the equipment before we go any further. You will be provided with pertinent information only when you ask the appropriate question. For any hands-on procedure, such as auscultation of a blood pressure or breath sounds or taking a pulse, select the appropriate equipment needed (if any) and use the equipment in the manner that it would be used on a patient. I will then give you the relevant clinical data. For example, you must select, place, and begin inflation of the BP cuff before the blood pressure is given to you. I will not answer questions in place of the patient. Therefore, it is imperative that you interact with your patient. Please verbalize to me any signs or symptoms that you find so that I will know you are cognizant of the patient and the patient's clinical appearance.

Scenario

Advise the participants that they are called to a residence for difficulty in breathing. When they arrive, they find a pale, extremely diaphoretic male (or female) patient pacing up and down the driveway. If the participants are nurses or in-hospital providers, the scenario can be modified to the medical environment—such as having the patient pull his or her car up to the front door of the ED and run to the triage desk, where the participants are sitting. The participants should use the assessment taught in this course.

Initial Impression: 28-year-old male (or female) suffering from acute difficulty in breathing.

Scene Size-up/General Impression: The scene is safe for entry and exit. There is no apparent injury on brief visual exam. The patient appears ill.

Initial Assessment:

Mental Status—Responsive and visibly agitated, alert and oriented to person, place, and time (A&O × 3)

Airway—Audible wheezes coming from patient with stridor

Breathing—Respirations rapid and shallow, breath sounds absent in the bases, wheezing in the apexes, very little air movement

Circulation—Radial pulse weak, skin cool and clammy

Disability—Moves all four extremities

Status after Initial Assessment: Serious, airway management initial concern.

Possible Differential (Field) Diagnoses: Exacerbation of asthma, respiratory infection, anaphylaxis, environmental emergency, acute bronchitis/pneumonia with bronchospasm. Encourage participants to share other possible etiologies.

Initial Management Priorities: High-flow oxygen at 15 lpm via NRM, IV access, blood glucose level, cardiac monitor, position of comfort.

Focused History (SAMPLE):

Signs and Symptoms—Agitated, audible airway sounds; decreased respiratory movement; weak radial pulses; cool and clammy extremities.

Allergies—Milk.

Medications—Patient denies any.

Past Medical History—Patient denies.

Last Oral Intake—This morning.

Events Preceding—Patient explains that he was cutting grass and felt a burning sensation in leg.

OPQRST:

Onset—Unknown; the patient is having extreme difficulty talking.

Palliation/Provocation—Worsens when the patient is placed in a supine position.

Quality—Unknown; the patient is having extreme difficulty talking.

Radiation—Unknown; the patient is having extreme difficulty talking.

Severity—If participants ask the patient if this reaction is worse than before, he will shake his head yes.

Time—Unknown; the patient is having extreme difficulty talking.

Vital Signs:

Respirations—34 with minimal chest rise and fall

Pulse—Radial pulse weak, barely palpable

Blood Pressure—98/palpation

Temperature—99.2°F (37.6°C)

Pulse Oximetry—92%

Blood Glucose Level—102 mg/dl (5.6 mmol/L)

Focused Physical Exam (Focused Medical Assessment): Raised erythematous patches (urticaria) to anterior chest and arms. Stinger visible at sting site.

Differential/Field Diagnosis: Distributive shock (anaphylactic reaction).

Management:

1) High-flow oxygen at 15 lpm via NRM; if insufficient respiratory movement, then PPV.

2) Remove antigen (e.g., stinger), being careful to avoid injecting additional venom.

3) Epinephrine 1:1,000 0.3–0.5 mg SQ (IV dose 0.1-0.5 mg of 1:10,000 for severe cardiovascular collapse).

4) IV access, fluid boluses to maintain 70–100 mmHg BP.

5) Diphenhydramine 10–25 mg IVP and steroid if available.

6) Inhaled bronchodilators if wheezing.

7) Cardiac monitor—sinus tachycardia with frequent premature ventricular contractions (PVCs).

8) Patient should be provided Epipen® before discharge.

Detailed Physical Exam: En route to receiving facility if time permits.

Ongoing Assessment: Continue to monitor respirations. Position patient for comfort.

Critical Actions:

1) Secure the airway and ensure highest oxygenation at 15 lpm via NRM.

2) If unstable airway, then PPV with RSI, if no severe airway swelling.

3) Maintain aggressive treatment with fluid bolus, epinephrine, and dopamine because of patient's condition. Emphasize that epinephrine is the critical treatment for anaphylaxis.

Teaching Points

1) There are numerous causes and etiologies of difficulty of breathing, and the focus should remain on assessment.

2) Always follow an organized approach to rule out possible causes.

3) Don't let past medical history lead you to a diagnosis preemptively.

4) Treatment priority is aggressive management to correct for cardiopulmonary collapse.

5) Abdominal cramping may occur from the smooth muscle contraction, vasodilation, and increased permeability.

6) Diphendydramine is a potent antihistamine that blocks H1 receptors that cause bronchoconstriction. Drugs like cimetidine and ranitidine block H2 receptors. These drugs are secondary to epinephrine because they are less effective at interrupting the major components of anaphylaxis (and have less impact on bronchospasm and vasodilation).

7) Explain the advantages and disadvantages of using an RSI.

Evaluation

1) *Excellent:* The participant's evaluation of the patient followed set format: initial assessment, focused history (SAMPLE, OPQRST) in an efficient manner. The participant displayed a thorough knowledge of the patient's condition, performed the exam and management in an organized manner, and demonstrated an excellent overall performance.

2) *Good:* The participant's evaluation of the patient followed set format: initial assessment, focused history (SAMPLE, OPQRST) in an acceptable manner with only minor deviation. The participant displayed an above-average knowledge of the patient's condition, performed the exam and management of the patient's condition, and demonstrated an above-average performance.

3) *Fair:* The participant's evaluation of the patient deviated from the set format without causing any further injury to the patient. The participant displayed an average or basic knowledge of the patient's condition and performed an adequate exam and management of the patient's condition.

4) *Inadequate:* The participant's evaluation of the patient deviated significantly from the set format, or the participant's actions endangered the patient's life or significantly exacerbated the condition.

DYSPNEA, RESPIRATORY DISTRESS, OR RESPIRATORY FAILURE

▶ DYSPNEA, RESPIRATORY DISTRESS, OR RESPIRATORY FAILURE: SCENARIO 1

Requirements: One instructor and one patient for every five participants.

Prerequisites: Read Chapter 5, "Dyspnea, Respiratory Distress, or Respiratory Failure."

Equipment: One table and chair for the patient to use; jump kit with oxygen supplies (NC, NRM, aerosol mask, PPV device, intubation equipment), stethoscope, BP cuff, cardiac monitor, pulse oximeter (optional but encouraged), and medication kit with associated medications

Instructor: Your role is vital because you must act as the coordinator of the station and also interact in the scenario. Before the participants arrive at the station, please review the scenario with your patient. For moulage, tint the patient's arms and face with a white coloring to simulate pale skin. Cheeks should be pinkish in color—use red coloring to simulate flushed cheeks. You will play the family of the patient, answering questions for the EMS providers about the condition of the patient. Please read the scenario to become familiar with the necessary responses. Encourage the participant to use the assessment format described during the assessment station with an emphasis on the SAMPLE and OPQRST history, and differential field diagnosis. Allow them to conduct the exam with minimal interruption or help.

Patient: One female (or male) patient. As the patient, you will be required to play the role of a 26-year-old female suffering from difficulty breathing. You will be awake and alert, but having trouble communicating verbally because of extreme difficulty breathing and a sore throat. You should breathe fast (at a rate of 24 per minute) and shallow, exaggerating your respiratory effort by using your diaphragm and neck muscles in an attempt to help you breathe. When you speak, you should speak with a quiet hoarse voice. When you answer questions, use as few words as possible and take breaths every few words. Please read the scenario to familiarize yourself with the information.

Instructions

Hi, my name is _____, and I will be the coordinator for this station. This is a hands-on patient assessment station. You will be given information concerning a patient experiencing a medical crisis. You will have all the necessary equipment you need to manage the patient in this station. Please look over the equipment before we go any further. You will be provided with pertinent information only when you ask the appropriate question. For any hands-on procedure, such as auscultation of a blood pressure or breath sounds or taking a pulse, select the appropriate equipment needed (if any) and use the equipment in the manner that it would be used on a patient. I will then give you the relevant clinical data. For example, you must select, place, and begin inflation of the BP cuff before the blood pressure is given to you. I will not answer questions in place of the patient. Therefore, it is imperative that you interact with your patient. Please verbalize to me any signs or symptoms that you find so that I will know you are cognizant of the patient and the patient's clinical appearance. The goal of this station is for you to complete an assessment with emphasis on use of the SAMPLE and OPQRST history to develop a differential field diagnosis and initiate appropriate treatment.

Scenario

Advise the participants that they are responding to an unknown medical emergency. If the participants are nurses or in-hospital providers, the scenario can be modified to the medical environment—such as the patient sitting in the triage chair. The participant should use the assessment taught in this course.

Initial Impression: 26-year-old female (or male) sitting in a chair in the living room (or at triage desk). She is sitting upright and leaning forward. The patient is awake, appears pale with cheeks flushed, and has accessory muscle usage.

Scene Size-up/General Impression: Family escorts you to the patient. The scene is safe for entry and exit. No injury is apparent on brief visual exam. Family members surround patient and are helpful with the history of events.

Initial Assessment:
Mental Status—Awake, obeys commands.

Airway—Open and patent; no C-spine precautions deemed necessary at this time.

Breathing—Respirations 24 and labored, accessory muscle usage noted in neck, diaphragmatic breathing noted, stridor noted on auscultation, remainder of lungs clear, patient speaks in a quiet hoarse voice.

Circulation—Rapid and strong—118 bpm

Disability/Perfusion—Moves all four extremities. Skin is flushed, pale, and warm.

Possible Differential (Field) Diagnoses: The following may be considered by the participants at this time: Upper airway problem such as foreign body obstruction, anaphylaxis, or infection (such as epiglottitis, peritonsilar abcess, or retropharyngeal abscess).

Status after Initial Assessment: Life threatening; needs immediate intervention.

Initial Management Priorities: High-flow oxygen at 15 lpm via NRM, be prepared for possible endotracheal intubation; cardiac monitor, IV access.

Focused History (SAMPLE):
Signs and Symptoms—Respiratory distress, tripod positioning, accessory muscle usage, hoarse voice.

NOTE: Either the family or the patient may answer the questions.

Allergies—Strawberries. If asked, the patient tells the providers she breaks out in hives and her chest feels a little tight when she eats strawberries. When this occurs, she takes diphenhydramine with relief.

Medications—Albuterol inhaler.

Past Medical History—Asthma.

Last Oral Intake—Breakfast. She does not believe she ate any strawberries, but cannot be sure.

Events Preceding—The patient has been sick and not feeling well for the last few days. She met some friends at a local restaurant this morning and ate from the buffet, but did not eat much because she was not feeling well.

OPQRST:

Onset—The problem began approximately 2 days ago, but the difficulty breathing has been getting progressively worse today.

Palliation/Provocation—Sitting up makes the breathing easier. It hurts to swallow and talk.

Quality—My throat feels tight and it hurts all the time.

Radiation—None.

Severity—An 8–9 on a 0–10 scale.

Time/Duration—The problem began approximately 2 days ago, but the difficulty breathing has been getting progressively worse today. The patient has never had an anaphylactic reaction or been intubated for her asthma.

Vital Signs:

Respirations—24 and labored

Pulse—Radial 118 bpm

Blood Pressure—128/76

Temperature—102°F (38.8°C)

Pulse Oximetry—97%

Blood Glucose Level—120 mg/dl (6.6 mmol/L)

Focused Physical Exam (Focused Medical Assessment): Rapid head-to-toe is unremarkable. Skin is warm to touch. Neck stiffness is noted. The remainder of the neurological exam is negative. Lungs are clear in the bases; stridor present on auscultation. Large abscess noted to the back of the throat on right side if mouth examined.

Differential/Field Diagnosis: Peritonsillar abscess.

Management:

1) High-flow oxygen at 15 lpm via NRM, humidified if possible.

2) Prepare for possible intubation. Airway may be shifted due to abscess. Avoid intubation or airway devices if at all possible—consider this difficult airway. Especially hazardous if epiglotitis.

3) Prepare for a possible needle or surgical cricothyrotomy.

4) Cardiac monitor—sinus tachycardia with no ectopy.

5) IV access at a moderate rate.

6) If patient deteriorates, PPV and endotracheal intubation with RSI:

    a) Sedative—midazolam 0.05–0.1 mg/kg IVP, diazepam 0.2 mg/kg IVP, etomidate 0.3 mg/kg, fentanyl 3–5 mcg/kg, or any of the other sedatives

    b) Cricoid pressure

c) Succinylcholine 1.5 mg/kg IVP

d) Intubation

e) Confirmation

7) Transport

Detailed Physical Exam: En route to appropriate facility as time permits.

Ongoing Assessment: Continue to monitor respiratory status. Maintain position of comfort.

Critical Actions:

1) Administer supplemental oxygen before beginning the focused examination. If supplemental oxygen is not applied or not applied in a high concentration (NRM above 12 lpm), then the patient's status should deteriorate—into increasing respiratory distress, the patient does not go into respiratory arrest.

2) Allow patient to maintain position of preference; avoid deep airway manipulation.

Teaching Points

1) Discuss the appearance of patients with difficulty breathing—leaning forward and the tripod position help facilitate increased respiratory expansion.

2) Ensure appropriate questioning of the respiratory patient.

3) Discuss the signs of respiratory difficulties—increased respiratory rate and effort, accessory muscle usage, stridor, increased pulse and hoarse voice.

4) Don't let past medical history lead you to a diagnosis preemptively.

5) Discuss treatment priorities—early use of high-flow oxygen via NRM, recognition of the possible need for PPV and intubation—because the patient can deteriorate rapidly. Discuss the use of RSI to help facilitate endotracheal intubation. Be prepared for surgical or needle cricocthyrotomy because airway may be distorted from edema and abscess. Due to potential difficult airway, it may be best to defer intubation until more resources available, such as anesthesia, ENT.

6) Discuss why this patient is most likely presenting abscess with a retropharyngeal abscess.

▶ Exam noted abscess on right—thus peritonsillar abscess likely. This is rare in aduts.

▶ Retropharyngeal abscess patients should be treated gently but aggressively. Patients with retropharyngeal abscess have up to a 50% mortality rate. Oxygen, IV fluids, and antibiotics are the treatment of choice. This patient most likely has an infectious disease—retropharyngeal abscess (fever, slow onset, stiff neck, sore throat, difficulty swallowing, and large abscess to back of throat).

▶ Is probably not presenting with

  ▶ anaphylaxis because the patient has a fever and slow onset. The patient does not have hives or other respiratory symptoms common to anaphylaxis.

  ▶ asthma because the patient does not have chest tightness. The patient has clear breath sounds with no wheezes. The patient is presenting with stridor instead.

  ▶ Foreign body obstruction because the patient has a fever and slow onset and an abscess.

  ▶ It is important to consider each of these possibilities because they are common presentations and require immediate intervention in the patient with respiratory distress.

Evaluation

1) *Excellent:* The participant's evaluation of the patient followed set format: initial assessment, focused history (SAMPLE, OPQRST) in an efficient manner. The participant displayed a thorough knowledge of the patient's condition, performed the exam and management in an organized manner, identified appropriate differential field diagnoses and demonstrated an excellent overall performance.

2) *Good:* The participant's evaluation of the patient followed set format: initial assessment, focused history (SAMPLE, OPQRST) in an acceptable manner with only minor deviation. The participant displayed an above-average knowledge of the patient's condition, performed the exam and management of the patient's condition, and demonstrated an above-average performance.

3) *Fair:* The participant's evaluation of the patient deviated from the set format without causing any further injury to the patient. The participant displayed an average or basic knowledge of the patient's condition and performed an adequate exam and management of the patient's condition.

4) *Inadequate:* The participant's evaluation of the patient deviated significantly from the set format, or the participant's actions endangered the patient's life or significantly exacerbated the condition.

▶ DYSPNEA, RESPIRATORY DISTRESS, OR RESPIRATORY FAILURE: SCENARIO 2

Requirements: One instructor and one patient for every five participants.

Prerequisites: Read Chapter 5, "Dyspnea, Respiratory Distress, or Respiratory Failure."

Equipment: One table and chair for the patient to use; jump kit with oxygen supplies (NC, NRM, aerosol mask, PPV device, intubation equipment), stethoscope, BP cuff, cardiac monitor, pulse oximeter (optional but encouraged), and medication kit with associated medications.

Instructor: Your role is vital because you must act as the coordinator of the station and also interact in the scenario. Before the participants arrive at the station, please review the scenario with your patient. For moulage, the patient should dress like an elderly male (female). The patient should try to keep his face as flaccid and expressionless as possible. His eyelids should be droopy and he or she cannot smile or lift his or her eyebrows. The patient is weak and can move only slightly and has very shallow breathing. He or she would not have signs of accessory muscle use because the muscles are too weak. Please read the scenario to become familiar with the necessary responses. Encourage the participants to use the assessment format described during the assessment station with an emphasis on the SAMPLE and OPQRST history, and differential field diagnosis. Allow them to conduct the exam with minimal interruption or help.

Patient: One male (or female) patient. As the patient, you will be required to play the role of a 64-year-old male or female suffering from difficulty breathing. You will be awake, confused, and anxious and able to communicate, but your voice will be very weak. Your respiratory rate will be 32 breaths per minute and shallow. You should keep your face as expressionless as possible. Keep your eyes droopy and do not smile or lift your eyebrows. You are weak and can move only slightly. Please read the scenario to familiarize yourself with all the information.

Instructions

Hi, my name is _____, and I will be the instructor for this station. This is a hands-on patient assessment station. You will be given information concerning a patient experiencing a medical crisis. You will have all the necessary equipment you need to manage the patient in this station. Please look over the equipment before we go any further. You will be provided with pertinent information only when you ask the appropriate question. For any hands-on procedure, such as auscultation of a blood pressure or breath sounds or taking a pulse, select the appropriate equipment needed (if any) and use the equipment in the manner that it would be used on a patient. I will then give you the relevant clinical data. For example, you must select, place, and begin inflation of the BP cuff before the blood pressure is given to you. I will not answer questions in place of the patient. Therefore, it is imperative that you interact with your patient. Please verbalize to me any signs or symptoms that you find so that I will know you are cognizant of the patient and the patient's clinical appearance. The goal of this station is for you to complete as assessment with emphasis on use of the AMPLE and OPQRST history to develop a differential field diagnosis and initiate appropriate treatment.

Scenario

Advise the participants that they are responding to a call for difficulty in breathing. If the participants are nurses or in-hospital providers, the scenario can be modified to the medical environment—such as EMS brings an elderly man to triage for evaluation. The participant should use the assessment taught in this course.

Initial Impression: 64-year-old ill-looking elderly male (or female).

Scene Size-up/General Impression: A family member escorts you to the patient. The scene is safe for entry and exit. No injury is apparent on brief visual exam.

Initial Assessment:

Mental Status—Awake, confused, weakly attempts to obey commands.

Airway—Open and patent

Breathing—Respirations 32 and shallow, breath sounds diminished with crackles throughout. Unable to take a deep breath if asked. No accessory muscle use.

Circulation—Radial pulse weak, irregular at 122 bpm, skin warm and dry to touch.

Disability/Perfusion—Moves all four extremities weakly. Skin is warm and dry.

Initial Field Diagnosis: The following may be considered by the students at this time: pneumonia, stroke, hypoglycemia, sepsis (others may be appropriate), ventilatory failure due to acute muscle weakness, or CNS condition.

Status after Initial Assessment: Potentially life threatening, unstable.

Initial Management Priorities: Oxygen at 10–15 liters via NRB, cardiac monitor, IV access.

Focused History (SAMPLE):

Signs and Symptoms—Respiratory distress, weak cough, and a fever.

Allergies—None.

Medications—Pyridostigmine, Prednisone.

Past Medical History—Myasthenia gravis, diabetes he controls with diet, and a recent history of TIAs (transient ischemic attacks).

Last Oral Intake—Unknown

Events Preceding—Family tells you the patient has not been feeling well for the last few days. Family member called to check on the patient this morning and did not get an answer. When family member arrived at the house, he found the patient in bed having trouble breathing and moving. If asked, the family member reports this is new to the patient.

OPQRST:

Onset—It started about two days ago.

Palliation/Provocation—Nothing, I just can't breathe.

Quality—I can't take a deep breath.

Radiation—None.

Severity—I don't have any energy; I feel worn out.

Time/Duration—I've been sick, but the breathing problem came on in the last few hours and is getting worse.

Vital Signs:

Respirations—32 and weak and shallow.

Pulse—Radial pulse irregular at 122 bpm. Monitor shows atrial fibrillation. Family is unsure about previous atrial fibrillation history. No jugular venous distension.

Blood Pressure—114/62.

Temperature—101.4°F (38.9°C).

Pulse Oximetry—93%.

Blood Glucose Level—98 mg/dl (5.4 mmol/L).

Focused Physical Exam (Focused Medical Assessment): The secondary assessment is negative. The patient has weak movement of all extremities. He obeys commands.

Differential/Field Diagnoses: Exacerbation of myasthenia gravis affecting respiratory ability, pneumonia/sepsis, possible stroke, pulmonary emboli, toxic inhalation, congestive heart failure.

Management:

1) Emotional reassurance to gain patient's confidence.

2) Oxygen by nasal cannula at 2–4 lpm or may select NRB with 10–15 lpm as the scenario progresses, breathing should become weaker and pulse oximetry deteriorates to 90% with oxygen—BVM assist or intubation should be considered.

3) Cardiac monitor.

4) IV access—possible rehydration if protocol allows.

Detailed Physical Exam: En route to appropriate facility if time permits.

Ongoing Assessment: As the scenario continues, respirations continue to weaken.

Critical Actions: Recognition of the patient's deteriorating respiratory status, specifically of inadequate ventilation (air exchange).

Teaching Points

1) Discuss the appearance of patients with respiratory compromise— mild versus severe. Discuss ventilatory compromise (air exchange) versus problems with oxygenation.

2) Ensure appropriate questioning of the respiratory patient.

3) Discuss the signs of respiratory difficulties—increased respiratory rate, weak respiratory effort, crackles.

4) Don't let past medical history lead you to a diagnosis preemptively.

5) Discuss treatment priorities—early use of oxygen and frequent re-evaluation of respiratory status with assistance of ventilations.

6) Discuss why this patient should be treated aggressively.

  ▶ Patients with myasthenia gravis may present with a weakening of the respiratory muscles when ill and rapidly deteriorate. Close monitoring of the respiratory status and assisting ventilation may be indicated. Lowering their temperature to normal when a fever is present may help as well.

7) Discuss the possible differential/field diagnoses.

  ▶ Exacerbation of myasthenia gravis (sudden onset of general weakness that has come on with illness in a patient with known myasthenia gravis).

  ▶ *Pneumonia/sepsis*—possible due to fever and crackles throughout lungs especially with weak respiratory effort of myasthenia gravis. (This patient has not had weakness until ill, but still possible.)

  ▶ *Possible stroke*—possible especially with atrial fibrillation, but not likely due to generalized weakness and weakness not isolated to one side.

  ▶ *Pulmonary emboli*—possible due to sudden onset, but crackles are not usually throughout the lungs.

  ▶ *Toxic inhalation*—important to rule out especially with generalized weakness and crackles, but no history of exposure in this patient.

  ▶ *Congestive heart failure*—possible, but EKG negative for infarct or left side enlargement and no previous cardiac history.

  ▶ *Hypoglycemia*—Blood sugar is within normal limits, but continued monitoring should be considered.

8) If RSI considered, vecuronium should be the paralytic of choice. Succinlycholine onset of action and duration is unpredictable in myasthenia gravis.

Evaluation

1) *Excellent:* The participant's evaluation of the patient followed set format: initial assessment, focused history (SAMPLE, OPQRST) in an efficient manner. The participant displayed a thorough knowledge of the patient's condition, performed the exam and management in an organized manner, identified appropriate differential field diagnoses and demonstrated an excellent overall performance.

2) *Good:* The participant's evaluation of the patient followed set format: initial assessment, focused history (SAMPLE, OPQRST) in an acceptable manner with only minor deviation. The participant displayed an above-average knowledge of the patient's condition, performed the exam and management of the patient's condition, and demonstrated an above-average performance.

3) *Fair:* The participant's evaluation of the patient deviated from the set format without causing any further injury to the patient. The participant displayed an average or basic knowledge of the patient's condition and performed an adequate exam and management of the patient's condition.

4) *Inadequate:* The participant's evaluation of the patient deviated significantly from the set format, or the participant's actions endangered the patient's life or significantly exacerbated the condition.

▶ Dyspnea, Respiratory Distress, or Respiratory Failure: Scenario 3

Requirements: One instructor and one patient for every five participants.

Prerequisites: Read Chapter 5, "Dyspnea, Respiratory Distress, or Respiratory Failure."

Equipment: One table and chair for the patient to use; jump kit with oxygen supplies (NC, NRM, aerosol mask, PPV device, intubation equipment), stethoscope, BP cuff, cardiac monitor, pulse oximeter (optional but encouraged), and medication kit with associated medications.

Instructor: Your role is vital because you must act as the coordinator of the station and also interact in the scenario. Before the participant arrives at the station, please review the scenario with your patient. For moulage, tint the patient's arms and face with a blue coloring to simulate cyanosis. Then spray the patient's arms with a fine mist of cool water to simulate cool and clammy skin. Please read the scenario to become familiar with the necessary responses. Do not "coach" the participants along during the testing station; rather, allow them to conduct the exam without interruption or help.

Patient: One male (or female) patient. As the patient, you will be required to play the role of a 28-year-old male suffering from difficulty in breathing (DIB). You will be awake and alert and able to communicate in short sentences. You should breathe fast (at a rate of 28 per minute) and shallow, exaggerating your respiratory effort by using your diaphragm and neck muscles in an attempt to help you breathe. To make the scenario as realistic as possible, cough frequently, attempting to clear out your airway. You will have a fine mist of cold water sprayed onto your arms and face by the instructor to simulate diaphoresis. Remember that you are short of breath, so you need to answer questions in short, broken sentences, pausing often to catch your breath. You were traveling with your family when you suddenly became short of breath. You have been driving for about 6 hours. Your chest is tight and it is difficult to breathe. You have a past history of asthma. Please read the scenario to familiarize yourself with the information.

Instructions

Hi, my name is _____, and I will be the instructor for this station. This is a hands-on patient assessment station. You will be given information concerning a patient experiencing a medical crisis. You will have all the necessary equipment you need to manage the patient in this station. Please look over the equipment before we go any further. You will be provided with pertinent information only when you ask the appropriate question. For any hands-on procedure, such as auscultation of a blood pressure or breath sounds or taking a pulse, select the appropriate equipment needed (if any) and use the equipment in the manner that it would be used on a patient. I will then give you the relevant clinical data. For example, you must select, place, and begin inflation of the BP cuff before the blood pressure is given to you. I will not answer questions in place of the patient. Therefore, it is imperative that you interact with your patient. Please verbalize to me any signs or symptoms that you find so that I will know you are cognizant of the patient and the patient's clinical appearance. The goal of this station is for you to complete as assessment with emphasis on use of the SAMPLE and OPQRST history to develop a differential field diagnosis and initiate appropriate treatment.

Scenario

Advise the participants that they are responding to a call for shortness of breath. You will find the patient seated in a vehicle. If the participants are nurses or in-hospital providers, the scenario can be modified to the medical environment—such as the triage nurse brings a patient who is short of breath to Medical Room 1. The participant should use the assessment taught in this course.

Initial Impression: Thin 28-year-old male (or female) sitting up and in obvious respiratory distress. The patient is awake, very anxious, appears cyanotic, and has accessory muscle usage.

Scene Size-up/General Impression: The scene is safe for entry and exit. No injury is apparent on brief visual exam.

Initial Assessment:

Mental Status—Awake, obeys commands, anxious.

Airway—Patent.

Breathing—Patient unable to talk in complete sentences, respirations 28 and shallow, accessory muscle usage noted in neck, diaphragmatic breathing noted, lung sounds in the bases absent with wheezes in the apices.

Circulation—Radial pulse regular at 108 bpm, skin cool and clammy. Pulse is more difficult to palpate when patient takes a deep breath.

Disability/Perfusion—Moves all four extremities. Skin is cool and clammy and patient presents with cyanosis on the lips.

Status after Initial Assessment: Potentially life threatening.

Possible Differential (Field) Diagnoses: The following may be considered by the participants at this time: asthma, anaphylaxis, spontaneous pneumothorax (others may be appropriate), upper airway or tracheal obstruction, pulmonary embolism, pneumonia, pleural effusion, toxio inhalation.

Initial Management Priorities: High-flow oxygen at 15 lpm via NRM, cardiac monitor, IV access, position of comfort, and bronchodilator nebulizer (Albuterol) reasonable choice at this time as well.

Focused History (SAMPLE):

Signs and Symptoms—Respiratory distress, leaning forward, accessory muscle usage, inability to speak in complete sentences.

Allergies—Grass, pollen, bees, penicillin.

Medications—Albuterol (Ventolin) inhaler. Used one time about 10 minutes ago without relief.

Past Medical History—Asthma, anaphylaxis to bee stings.

Last Oral Intake—Soda and chips about an hour ago.

Events Preceding—Began to have mild difficulty breathing while traveling in the car. The patient developed an inability to breathe that was almost suffocating. The patient opened the window to let in some air and his breathing became even worse. The driver pulled the car to the side of the road to assist the patient with his inhaler and called EMS.

OPQRST:

Onset—I've been mildly short of breath for the past few days, and it got worse this evening.

Palliation/Provocation—When I sit forward, it feels as if I can catch my breath. If I lie back, I feel like I'm suffocating.

Quality—It feels like I'm suffocating, like my chest is being squeezed.

Radiation—None, just the tightness in my lungs.

Severity—I can't even talk without becoming winded. I can't remember it ever being this bad this fast.

Time/Duration—It came on suddenly—about 10–15 minutes ago. (If the participants ask about past episodes of respiratory failure and whether or not the patient has ever had to be intubated before, the reply will be almost when he had his anaphylactic reaction to the last bee sting. The patient does not believe he was stung at this time, and there is no evidence of a bee sting.)

Vital Signs:

Respirations—28 and labored and shallow.

Pulse—Radial pulse regular at 108 bpm, skin cool and clammy. Pulse is more difficult to palpate when patient takes a deep breath. EKG is negative. Monitor shows sinus tachycardia.

Blood Pressure—112/78.

Temperature—98.8°F (37.1°C).

Pulse Oximetry—91%.

Blood Glucose Level—128 mg/dl (7.1 mmol/L).

Focused Physical Exam (Focused Medical Assessment): Peripheral cyanosis that is getting worse.

Differential/Field Diagnosis: Exacerbation of asthma.

Management:

1) High-flow oxygen at 15 lpm via NRM

3) Cardiac monitor—sinus tachycardia

4) IV access

5) Nebulized albuterol (or other beta 2–specific medication) 2.5 mg treatment

6) If patient deteriorates, then PPV and endotracheal intubation with RSI:

   a) Defasciculating agent—vecuronium 0.01 mg/kg IVP

   b) Sedative—midazolam 0.05–0.1 mg/kg IVP, diazepam 0.2 mg/kg IVP, fentanyl 3–5 mcg/kg, or any of the other sedatives

   c) Cricoid pressure

   d) Succinylcholine 1.5 mg/kg IVP

   e) Intubation

   f) Confirmation

Detailed Physical Exam: En route to appropriate facility as time permits.

Ongoing Assessment: Continue to monitor respiratory status. Maintain position of comfort.

Critical Actions:

1) Administer supplemental oxygen before beginning the focused examination. If supplemental oxygen is not applied or not applied in a high concentration (NRM above 12 lpm), then the patient's status should deteriorate into respiratory arrest.

2) If the participants base their actions on the pulse oximeter reading without any correlation to the patient's signs or symptoms, the patient should deteriorate into respiratory arrest.

Teaching Points

1) Discuss the appearance of patients with difficulty breathing—leaning forward.

2) Ensure appropriate questioning of the respiratory patient.

3) Discuss the signs of respiratory difficulties—increased respiratory rate and effort, accessory muscle usage, breath sounds and adventitious sounds, increased pulse and BP, pulsus paradoxus, pulse oximetry reading, and inability to talk in complete sentences.

4) Don't let past medical history lead you to a diagnosis preemptively.

5) Discuss treatment priorities—early use of high-flow oxygen via NRM, recognition of the possible need for PPV and intubation—because the patient can deteriorate rapidly. Discuss the use of RSI to help facilitate endotracheal intubation.

6) Review the indications for fluid resuscitation and other medications such as subcutaneous epinephrine (age consideration), inhaled anticholinergics, coritcosteroids and magnesium sulfate, or other asthma management pharmacological tools. CPAP/BiPAP and Heliox should be considered as well.

7) Discuss the possible differential/field diagnoses.

   ▶ Exacerbation of asthma (sudden onset of respiratory distress and wheezing in a patient with known asthma history).

   ▶ Anaphylactic reaction—possible due to sudden onset, wheezing, previous history, but not as likely because no evidence of exposure.

   ▶ Possible pulmonary emboli—possible especially with sudden onset and long driving time. Not as likely due to lack of other contributing history and wheezing bilateral and diminished breath sounds bilateral.

   ▶ Spontaneous pneumothorax—possible due to sudden onset and patient presentation (thin male or female), but breath sounds the same on both sides.

   ▶ Toxic inhalation—important to rule out especially with respiratory distress and wheezes, but no history of exposure in this patient or signs and symptoms in other passengers.

Evaluation

1) *Excellent:* The participant's evaluation of the patient followed set format: initial assessment, focused history (SAMPLE, OPQRST) in an efficient manner. The participant displayed a thorough knowledge of the patient's condition, performed the exam and management in an organized manner, identified appropriate differential field diagnoses and demonstrated an excellent overall performance.

2) *Good:* The participant's evaluation of the patient followed set format: initial assessment, focused history (SAMPLE, OPQRST) in an acceptable manner with only minor deviation. The participant displayed an above-average knowledge of the patient's condition, performed the exam and management of the patient's condition, and demonstrated an above-average performance.

3) *Fair:* The participant's evaluation of the patient deviated from the set format without causing any further injury to the patient. The participant displayed an average or basic knowledge of the patient's condition and performed an adequate exam and management of the patient's condition.

4) *Inadequate:* The participant's evaluation of the patient deviated significantly from the set format, or the participant's actions endangered the patient's life or significantly exacerbated the condition.

▶ DYSPNEA, RESPIRATORY DISTRESS, OR RESPIRATORY FAILURE: SCENARIO 4

Requirements: One instructor and one patient for every five participants.

Prerequisites: Read Chapter 5, "Dyspnea, Respiratory Distress, or Respiratory Failure."

Equipment: One table and chair for the patient to use; jump kit with oxygen supplies (NC, NRM, aerosol mask, PPV device, intubation equipment), stethoscope, BP cuff, cardiac monitor, pulse oximeter (optional but encouraged), and medication kit with associated medications

Instructor: Your role is vital because you must act as the coordinator of the station and also interact in the scenario. Before the participants arrive at the station, please review the scenario with your patient. For moulage, tint the patient's arms and face with a blue coloring to simulate cyanosis. Then spray the patient's arms with a fine mist of cool water to simulate cool and clammy skin. Please read the scenario to become familiar with the necessary responses. Do not "coach" the participants along during the testing station; rather, allow them to conduct the exam without interruption or help.

Patient: One female (or male) patient. As the patient, you will be required to play the role of a 78-year-old female suffering from difficulty in breathing (DIB). You will be sleepy and difficult to arouse and able to communicate in short sentences. You should breathe slow (at a rate of 8-10 per minute) and shallow, exaggerating your respiratory effort by using your diaphragm and neck muscles in an attempt to help you breathe. You will have a fine mist of cold water sprayed onto your arms and face by the instructor to simulate cool, clammy skin. The instructor will act as your son or daughter. Initially, you answer only to yes and no questions with stimulus. After you are administered narcan you can answer additional questions. If questioned about the history behind the mild DIB, you will answer that you had mild DIB before bedtime. You woke very anxious and moderately short of breath with chest discomfort. You took your Tylenol #3 for pain. When the pain did not stop, you took two more of your pain pills and then you don't remember anything else. You always sleep with two pillows under your back. You have had two past myocardial infarctions. You currently take digoxin (Lanoxin), furosemide (Lasix), prazosin (Minipress), and potassium supplements (Kaochlor), Prozac for depression, and Tylenol #3 for pain after recent hip surgery. If questioned, after you are awake, about when you last took your medications, hesitantly reply that you ran out of your water pill two weeks ago and haven't had the money to refill it since. Remember that you are short of breath, so you need to answer questions in short, broken sentences, pausing often to catch your breath. Please read the scenario to familiarize yourself with the information.

Instructions

Hi, my name is _____, and I will be the instructor for this station. This is a hands-on patient assessment station. You will be given information concerning a patient experiencing a medical crisis. You will have all the necessary equipment you need to manage the patient in this station. Please look over the equipment before we go any further. You will be provided with pertinent information only when you ask the appropriate question. For any hands-on procedure, such as auscultation of a blood pressure or breath sounds or taking a pulse, select the appropriate equipment needed (if any) and use the equipment in the manner that it would be used on a patient. I will then give you the relevant clinical data. For example, you must select, place, and begin inflation of the BP cuff before the blood pressure is given to you. I will not answer questions in place of the patient. Therefore, it is imperative that you interact with your patient. Please verbalize to me any signs or symptoms that you find so that I will know you are cognizant of the patient and the patient's clinical appearance. The goal of this station is for you to complete an assessment with emphasis on use of the AMPLE and OPQRST history to develop a differential field diagnosis and initiate appropriate treatment.

Scenario

Advise the participants that they are responding to a call of difficulty in breathing at a residence. If the participants are nurses or in-hospital providers, the scenario can be modified to the medical environment—such as the triage nurse brings a patient who has difficulty breathing to Medical Room 1. The participant should use the assessment taught in this course.

Initial Impression: 78-year-old female (or male) sitting in bed at home or in ED, with two to three pillows propped up behind her. The patient is very sleepy, appears pale with circumoral cyanosis, and has accessory muscle usage.

Scene Size-up/General Impression: The scene is safe for entry and exit. No injury is apparent on brief visual exam.

Initial Assessment:
Mental Status—Somnolent (continues to fall asleep), arouses to pain, and obeys commands when stimulated then falls back to sleep when stimulus stops.

Airway—Patent.

Breathing—Respirations 10 and shallow, accessory muscle usage noted in neck, diaphragmatic breathing noted, lung sounds crackle throughout.

Circulation—Radial pulse regular and 120 bpm, skin cool and clammy.

Disability/Perfusion—Moves all four extremities. Skin is cool and clammy.

Status after Initial Assessment: Serious, potentially life threatening.

Possible Differential (Field) Diagnoses: The following may be considered by the participants at this time: CHF, Acute Coronary Syndrome, stroke, CNS event, toxicology syndrome, pneumonia, COPD exacacerbated by hypoxia/CO_2 retention (others may be appropriate).

Initial Management Priorities: High-flow oxygen at 15 lpm via NRM, cardiac monitor, IV access, position of comfort.

Focused History (SAMPLE):
Signs and Symptoms—Respiratory depression, sitting up with pillows behind her or him, accessory muscle usage, inability to speak in complete sentences. Extremely sleepy. Circumoral and peripheral cyanosis.

Allergies—No known food or drug allergies.

Medications—Lanoxin, Lasix, Minipress, Kaochlor, Prozac, Tylenol #3

Past Medical History—Two previous MIs and a hip replacement 3 weeks ago.

Last Oral Intake—Dinner 3-4 hours ago.

Events Preceding—Initially, information can be obtained only from the son. Her son came in to check on her before going to bed and found her with slurred speech and hard to awaken so he called EMS. If narcan is administered to the patient, the following information may be obtained. The patient began to have mild trouble before going to bed. The patient awoke with an inability to breathe that was almost suffocating. Then the patient began having chest pain, so she took the pain medication the doctor gave her for her hip. She remembers taking them at least one or two more times.

OPQRST:

Onset—Son found her right before he called you, which is about 10 minutes ago. Last saw his mother normal just after dinner 3–4 hours ago. She had gone to lie down in her room because she wasn't feeling well.

Palliation/Provocation—Patient wakes up and breathes a little deeper with stimulus.

Quality—Poor respiratory effort.

Radiation—None.

Severity—After narcan, she reports the discomfort and respiratory distress to be a 7–8 on the pain scale.

Time/Duration—Son found her right before he called you, which is about 10 minutes ago. Last saw his mother normal just after dinner 3–4 hours ago. She had gone to lie down in her room because she wasn't feeling well. When patient is awake, she tells you the pain started shortly after she went to bed. When asked about medications will tell you she has not taken her Lasix (water pill) for two weeks because she ran out of money and has not been able to get it refilled.

Vital Signs:

Respirations—10 and shallow.

Pulse—Radial pulse 120 bpm, skin cool and clammy, EKG show sinus tachycardia, 12 lead shows ST elevation in V1, V2, V3, V4, and Q waves in V3 and V4.

Blood Pressure—156/94.

Temperature—97.8°F (36.5°).

Pulse Oximetry—92%.

Blood Glucose Level—118 mg/dl (6.5 mmol/L).

Focused Physical Exam (Focused Medical Assessment): Bilateral 3+ pitting edema to the ankles; pinpoint pupils.

Differential/Field Diagnosis: Congestive heart failure with acute pulmonary edema, acute coronary syndrome, possible acute ST elevation MI, narcotic overdose, pulmonary emboli, stroke, toxic exposure.

Management:

1) High-flow oxygen at 15 lpm via NRM.

2) Cardiac monitor—sinus tachycardia, 12 lead shows ST elevation in V1, V2, V3, V4, and Q waves in V3 and V4.

3) IV access.

4) Narcan 0.4–2 mg IVP or IM.

5) Nitroglycerin sublingual 0.4 mg or nitroglycerin drip as protocol allows.

6) Lasix 0.5–1.0 mg/kg IVP.

7) Aspirin 160–325 mg po chewed after patient is awake.

Detailed Physical Exam: En route to appropriate facility as time permits.

Ongoing Assessment: Continue to monitor for respiratory distress or decreasing level of consciousness. Maintain position of comfort.

Critical Actions:

1) Administer supplemental oxygen before beginning the focused examination. If supplemental oxygen is not applied or not applied in a high concentration (NRM above 12 lpm), then the patient's status should deteriorate. Consider need for PPV.

2) If the participants bases their actions on the pulse oximeter reading without any correlation to the patient's signs or symptoms, the patient should deteriorate.

Teaching Points

1) Discuss the appearance of patients with DIB—using multiple pillows to sleep, decreased level of consciousness and slowing shallow respiratory rate, and crackles.

2) Discuss the appearance of peripheral versus central cyanosis.

3) Ensure appropriate questioning of the respiratory patient and family.

4) Discuss the importance of medication history.

5) Don't let past medical history lead you to a diagnosis preemptively.

6) Discuss treatment priorities—early use of high-flow oxygen via NRM, recognition of the possible need for PPV and intubation—because the patient can deteriorate rapidly. Discuss the use of RSI to help facilitate endotracheal intubation. Discuss the importance of narcan administration before intubation when altered level of consciousness is present.

   As part of the management for CHF—wherein the initial concern is to decrease preload and afterload—the best choice is NTG. Lasix should be considered only if peripheral edema or other signs of true volume overload (vs. acute fluid shift) are present. CPAP/BiPAP can help avoid intubation.

7) Discuss the possible differential/field diagnoses.

   ▶ Congestive heart failure with acute pulmonary edema—highly likely due to previous history, not taking medication, and presentation with wet lung sounds and pedal edema.

   ▶ Acute coronary syndrome—due to chest pain and EKG changes.

   ▶ Narcotic overdose—due to taking Tylenol with codeine for pain.

   ▶ Pulmonary emboli—possible due to recent surgery and not feeling well. Not as likely due to breath sounds and presentation.

▶ Stroke—should be considered due to altered level of consciousness, but not likely because no neurological deficit after the narcan is administered.

▶ Toxic exposure—should be considered due to decreased level of responsiveness and pulmonary edema. Not likely because no evidence of exposure and son has no effects.

Evaluation

1) *Excellent:* The participant's evaluation of the patient followed set format: initial assessment, focused history (SAMPLE, OPQRST) in an efficient manner. The participant displayed a thorough knowledge of the patient's condition, performed the exam and management in an organized manner, identified appropriate differential field diagnoses and demonstrated an excellent overall performance.

2) *Good:* The participant's evaluation of the patient followed set format: initial assessment, focused history (SAMPLE, OPQRST) in an acceptable manner with only minor deviation. The participant displayed an above-average knowledge of the patient's condition, performed the exam and management of the patient's condition, and demonstrated an above-average performance.

3) *Fair:* The participant's evaluation of the patient deviated from the set format without causing any further injury to the patient. The participant displayed an average or basic knowledge of the patient's condition and performed an adequate exam and management of the patient's condition.

4) *Inadequate:* The participant's evaluation of the patient deviated significantly from the set format, or the participant's actions endangered the patient's life or significantly exacerbated the condition.

⊞ CHEST DISCOMFORT OR PAIN

▶ CHEST DISCOMFORT: SCENARIO 1

Requirements: One instructor and one patient for every five participants.

Prerequisites: Read Chapter 6, "Chest Discomfort or Pain."

Equipment: One table and chair for the patient to use; jump kit with oxygen supplies (NC, NRM, aerosol mask, PPV device, intubation equipment), stethoscope, BP cuff, cardiac monitor, pulse oximeter (optional but encouraged), and medication kit with associated medications

Instructor: Your role is vital because you must act as the coordinator of the station and also interact in the scenario. Before the participants arrive at the station, please review the scenario with your patient. No moulage necessary. Please read the scenario to become familiar with the necessary responses. Encourage the participants to use the assessment format described during the assessment station with an emphasis on the SAMPLE and OPQRST history and differential field diagnosis. Allow them to conduct the exam with minimal interruption or help.

Patient: One female (or male) patient. As the patient, you will be required to play the role of a 33-year-old female (or male) suffering from chest pain. You started a new job that requires a lot of lifting; you have been a little stiff, but the pain has gotten so bad that you can't even take a deep breath. Please read the scenario to become familiar with the information.

Instructions

Hi, my name is _____, and I will be the coordinator for this station. This is a hands-on patient assessment station. You will be given information concerning a patient experiencing a medical crisis. You will have all the necessary equipment you need to manage the patient in this station. Please look over the equipment before we go any further. You will be provided with pertinent information only when you ask the appropriate question. For any hands-on procedure, such as auscultation of a blood pressure or breath sounds or taking a pulse, select the appropriate equipment needed (if any) and use the equipment in the manner that it would be used on a patient. I will then give you the relevant clinical data. For example, you must select, place, and begin inflation of the BP cuff before the blood pressure is given to you. I will not answer questions in place of the patient. Therefore, it is imperative that you interact with your patient. Please verbalize to me any signs or symptoms that you find so that I will know you are cognizant of the patient and the patient's clinical appearance. The goal of this station is for you to complete an assessment with emphasis on use of the SAMPLE and OPQRST history to develop a differential field diagnosis and initiate appropriate treatment.

Scenario

Advise the participants that they are responding to a call of chest pain. If the participants are nurses or in-hospital providers, the scenario can be modified to the medical environment—such as the patient walked into triage complaining of chest pain. The participant should use the assessment taught in this course.

Initial Impression: 33-year-old female (or male) sitting in a chair/triage desk leaning forward.

Scene Size-up/General Impression: You respond to a local grocery store. The scene is safe for entry and exit. No injury is apparent on brief visual exam. At the scene, you see a pallet of canned goods partially unloaded nearby.

Initial Assessment:
Mental Status—Responsive, A&O × 3, GCS 15.

Airway—Open and clear.

Breathing—Respirations 14 and regular, breath sounds equal, slightly decreased in the bases due to shallow breathing.

Circulation—Radial pulse regular 72 bpm. Skin warm, dry, and pink.

Disability/Perfusion—Moves all extremities to command. Skin warm, dry, and pink.

Status after Initial Assessment: Serious, Not life-threatening.

Possible Differential (Field) Diagnoses: Angina/acute coronary syndrome, pulmonary emboli, pleurisy, spontaneous pneumothorax, chest wall pain, chostochondritis (muscle strain), others may be appropriate.

Initial Management Priorities: Oxygen as necessary, cardiac monitor, IV access, position of comfort.

Focused History (SAMPLE):
Signs and Symptoms—Chest pain with complaints of pain with breathing.

Allergies—NKA.

Medications—Patient denies any.

Past Medical History—Patient denies.

Last Oral Intake—About an hour ago, breakfast before coming to work.

Events Preceding—The patient explains that she or he was beginning to unload the pallet, when the pain became so bad she or he could not move any more boxes. It hurts even when she breathes.

OPQRST:
Onset—Gradual. She has been hurting since she took this job and now it hurts so bad she can't lift anything or even breathe.

Palliation/Provocation—It hurts when I try to lift the boxes or take a deep breath.

Quality—Sharp pain.

Radiation—No radiation.

Severity—On a scale of 1 to 10, it's a 7.

Time/Duration—Pain occurred when lifting the boxes and is not as noticeable since the patient rested.

Vital Signs:
Respirations—16 and regular.

Pulse—Radial pulse at 72 bpm.

Blood Pressure—126/82.

Temperature—99.2°F (37.6°C).

Pulse Oximetry—99%.

Blood Glucose Level—112 mg/dl (6.1 mmol/L).

Focused Physical Exam (Focused Medical Assessment): Rapid head-to-toe is unremarkable. Patient complains of pain if chest is palpated. Pain can be reproduced.

Differential/Field Diagnosis: Angina/acute coronary syndrome, pulmonary emboli, spontaneous pneumothorax, chostochondritis, pleurisy.

Management:

1) High-flow oxygen at 15 lpm via NRM.

2) IV access.

3) Cardiac monitor—sinus tachycardia with no ectopy, 12 lead ECG negative if done.

4) Transport to the appropriate facility.

5) Continue monitoring for changes in status, cardiac rhythm, breath sounds.

Critical Actions:

1) Secure airway and ensure highest oxygenation at 15 lpm via NRM.

2) Allow the patient to assume position of comfort for breathing.

3) Consider potential cardiac involvement.

Teaching Points

1) There are numerous causes and etiologies of chest pain. Assist the participants in classifying chest pain to body system and causes (e.g., cardiac vs. respiratory, trauma vs. medical) for rule outs.

2) Always follow an organized approach to rule out possible causes.

3) Compare and contrast clinical findings.

4) Discuss the possible differential/field diagnoses

   ▶ Angina/AMI—Possible due to history. Age of patient makes it less likely. It would be important to keep this potential diagnosis on the list because patients can have costrochondritis and an AMI. Even though the electrocardiogram (ECG) is negative, damage may still be a potential, so cardiac monitoring should be continued.

   ▶ Pulmonary emboli—Possible, but no identifiable risk factors, oxygen saturation remains good.

   ▶ Spontaneous pneumothorax—Possible, but unlikely due to equal breath sounds. Continue to monitor breath sounds.

   ▶ Chostochondritis or muscle strain—Very likely due to repetitive work and muscle use. Use diagnosis with caution and continue to monitor for lifethreats.

Evaluation

1) *Excellent:* The participant's evaluation of the patient followed set format: initial assessment, focused history (SAMPLE, OPQRST) in an efficient manner. The participant displayed a thorough knowledge of the patient's condition, performed the exam and management in an organized manner, identified appropriate differential field diagnoses and demonstrated an excellent overall performance.

2) *Good:* The participant's evaluation of the patient followed set format: initial assessment, focused history (SAMPLE, OPQRST) in an acceptable manner with only minor deviation. The participant displayed an above-average knowledge of the patient's condition, performed the exam and management of the patient's condition, and demonstrated an above-average performance.

3) *Fair:* The participant's evaluation of the patient deviated from the set format without causing any further injury to the patient. The participant displayed an average or basic knowledge of the patient's condition and performed an adequate exam and management of the patient's condition.

4) *Inadequate:* The participant's evaluation of the patient deviated significantly from the set format, or the participant's actions endangered the patient's life or significantly exacerbated the condition.

▶ CHEST DISCOMFORT: SCENARIO 2

> *Requirements:* One instructor and one patient for every five participants.
>
> *Prerequisites:* Read Chapter 6, "Chest Discomfort or Pain."
>
> *Equipment:* One table and chair for the patient to use; jump kit with oxygen supplies (NC, NRM, aerosol mask, PPV device, intubation equipment), stethoscope, BP cuff, cardiac monitor, pulse oximeter (optional but encouraged), and medication kit with associated medications

Instructor: Your role is vital because you must act as the coordinator of the station and also interact in the scenario. Before the participants arrive at the station, please review the scenario with your patient. You also will act as the family member. As the patient's respiratory distress worsens, you will need to provide the history. Please read the scenario to become familiar with the necessary responses. Encourage the participants to use the assessment format described during the assessment station with an emphasis on the SAMPLE and OPQRST history and differential field diagnosis. Allow them to conduct the exam with minimal interruption or help.

Patient: One male (or female) patient. As the patient, you will be required to play the role of a 74-year-old male (or female) suffering from chest pain. You will be awake and alert and able to answer all questions initially, but are having trouble breathing, so pause between words and get to the point that you can only nod yes and no. You are having respiratory distress and chest pain. The pain and distress are becoming more severe. You seem to get worse with each breath. You have a history of emphysema from years of smoking. Please read the scenario to become familiar with all the information.

Instructions

Hi, my name is _____, and I will be the coordinator for this station. This is a hands-on patient assessment station. You will be given information concerning a patient experiencing a medical crisis. You will have all the necessary equipment you need to manage the patient in this station. Please look over the equipment before we go any further. You will be provided with pertinent information only when you ask the appropriate question. For any hands-on procedure, such as auscultation of a blood pressure or breath sounds or taking a pulse, select the appropriate equipment needed (if any) and use the equipment in the manner that it would be used on a patient. I will then give you the relevant clinical data. For example, you must select, place, and begin inflation of the BP cuff before the blood pressure is given to you. I will not answer questions in place of the patient. Therefore, it is imperative that you interact with your patient. Please verbalize to me any signs or symptoms that you find so that I will know you are cognizant of the patient and the patient's clinical appearance. The goal of this station is for you to complete an assessment with emphasis on use of the SAMPLE and OPQRST history to develop a differential field diagnosis and initiate appropriate treatment.

Scenario

Advise the participants that they are responding to a home for a chest pain call. If the participants are nurses or in-hospital providers, the scenario can be modified to the medical environment—such as the patient has walked into the ED and collapsed in the triage seat. The participant should use the assessment taught in this course.

Initial Impression: 74-year-old male (or female) nursing home patient sitting in a chair.

Scene Size-up/General Impression: The scene is safe for entry and exit. No injury is apparent on brief visual exam. The family directs you to an elderly thin male patient. You see a full ashtray of cigarette butts next to the patient. The room has the smell of cigarette smoke when you arrive.

Initial Assessment:

Mental Status—Awake, alert, in distress, leaning forward to breathe.

Airway—Audible wheeze present.

Breathing—Respirations 32 and very labored. Pursed lip breathing. Tongue bright pink. If assessed, breath sounds decreased on the right.

Circulation—Radial pulse 104 bpm and irregular.

Disability/Perfusion—Moves all four extremities. Skin very warm and dry to touch. Nailbeds and lips cyanotic.

Status after Initial Assessment: Life threatening; immediate intervention required.

Possible Differential (Field) Diagnoses: COPD, pulmonary emboli, pneumonia, spontaneous pneumothorax, AMI/CHF, aortic dissection, cardiac tamponade, esophageal disruption.

Initial Management Priorities: High-flow oxygen at 15 lpm via NRM, cardiac monitor, IV access.

Focused History (SAMPLE):

Signs and Symptoms—Chest pain, difficulty breathing, skin warm to touch.

Allergies—Sulfa drugs.

Medications—Inhaler, prednisone, antibiotics for recent bout of pneumonia, antacid.

Past Medical History—COPD, arthritis, esophageal reflux, smokes two packs a day for at least 60 years.

Last Oral Intake—At lunchtime.

Events Preceding—The patient is recovering from pneumonia. He has been on antibiotics for five days and was doing better. He had an episode of coughing and is having pain and trouble breathing. The coughing is normal for him.

OPQRST:

Onset—He is always a little short of breath, but not like this. This started right before they called you—10 minutes maximum.

Palliation/Provocation—I can't get my breath. Nothing helps.

Quality—Just can't breathe.

Radiation—None.

Severity—On a scale of 1 to 10, it's a 10.

Time/Duration—Pneumonia one week. The chest pain and distress has been occurring for approximately 10 minutes.

Vital Signs:

    Respirations—32 and labored

    Pulse—Radial pulse weak, rapid and irregular at 104 bpm

    Blood Pressure—100/67

    Temperature—96.6°F (35.8°C)

    Pulse Oximetry—87%

    Blood Glucose Level—138 mg/dl

Focused Physical Exam (Focused Medical Assessment): Distended neck veins, decreased breath sounds on the right. Wheezes throughout the remainder of his lungs.

Differential/Field Diagnosis: Pneumothorax

Management:

  1) Supplemental oxygen at 15 lpm via NRM.

  2) Chest decompression on the right – if done, the patient's breathing eases.

  3) IV access

  4) Cardiac monitor—artrial fibrillation; 12 lead shows right ventricular enlargement.

  5) Transport in position of comfort. Communicate with the receiving facility the need for a possible chest tube.

Critical Actions:

  1) Secure airway and ensure highest oxygenation at 15 lpm via NRM.

  2) Chest decompression or recognition of the need if unable to perform the skill.

  3) Do not force patient to lie on the cot.

Teaching Points

  1) There are numerous causes and etiologies of chest pain. Assist the participant in classifying chest pain to body system and causes (e.g., cardiac vs. respiratory, trauma vs. medical) for rule outs.

  2) Always follow an organized approach to rule out possible causes.

  3) Discuss the possible differential/field diagnoses.

    ▶ *COPD*—This is a COPD patient because he is a long-term smoker with respiratory presentation consistent with COPD, but his distress is not normal so the patient has some other problem causing his symptoms.

    ▶ *Pulmonary emboli*—Possible, the low oxygen saturation could indicate a pulmonary emboli, but the decreased breath sounds on one side are more consistent with another diagnosis.

    ▶ *Spontaneous pneumothorax*—Likely due to unequal breath sounds. His history of COPD and weakened lung tissue puts him at risk. The sudden onset after coughing makes this diagnosis more likely. A tension pneumothorax is most likely developing and decompression is indicated.

- *AMI/CHF*—Possible, but ECG is negative at this time, and breath sounds are unequal which is not consistent with each diagnosis. It would be important to keep this potential diagnosis on the list because this patient could still develop an AMI, so cardiac monitoring should be continued.

- *Aortic dissection*—Not likely due to presentation and respiratory involvement.

- *Cardiac tamponade*—Possible, but not likely due to pain description and respiratory involvement.

- *Pneumonia*—Probably still present, but not likely the cause of the acute onset of distress.

- *Esophageal disruption*—Possible due to reflux history and severe episode of coughing, but spontaneous pneumothorax more likely.

Evaluation

1) *Excellent:* The participant's evaluation of the patient followed set format: initial assessment, focused history (SAMPLE, OPQRST) in an efficient manner. The participant displayed a thorough knowledge of the patient's condition, performed the exam and management in an organized manner, identified appropriate differential field diagnoses and demonstrated an excellent overall performance.

2) *Good:* The participant's evaluation of the patient followed set format: initial assessment, focused history (SAMPLE, OPQRST) in an acceptable manner with only minor deviation. The participant displayed an above-average knowledge of the patient's condition, performed the exam and management of the patient's condition, and demonstrated an above-average performance.

3) *Fair:* The participant's evaluation of the patient deviated from the set format without causing any further injury to the patient. The participant displayed an average or basic knowledge of the patient's condition and performed an adequate exam and management of the patient's condition.

4) *Inadequate:* The participant's evaluation of the patient deviated significantly from the set format, or the participant's actions endangered the patient's life or significantly exacerbated the condition.

▶ CHEST DISCOMFORT: SCENARIO 3

Requirements: One instructor and one patient for every five participants.

Prerequisites: Read Chapter 6, "Chest Discomfort or Pain."

Equipment: One table and chair for the patient to use; jump kit with oxygen supplies (NC, NRM, aerosol mask, PPV device, intubation equipment), stethoscope, BP cuff, cardiac monitor, pulse oximeter (optional but encouraged), and medication kit with associated medications

Instructor: Your role is vital because you must act as the coordinator of the station and also interact in the scenario. Before the participants arrive at the station, please review the scenario with your patient. Spray the patient's arms with a fine mist of cool water to simulate cool and clammy skin. Please read the scenario to become familiar with the necessary responses. Do not "coach" the participants along during the testing station; rather, allow them to conduct the exam without interruption or help.

Patient: One female (or male) patient. As the patient, you will be required to play the role of a 46-year-old female (or male) suffering from chest pain. You will be awake and alert and clutching your chest because of the intense pain. Please read the scenario to become familiar with the information.

Instructions

Hi, my name is _____, and I will be the examiner for this station. This is a hands-on patient assessment station. You will be given information concerning a patient experiencing a medical crisis. You will have all the necessary equipment you need to manage the patient in this station. Please look over the equipment before we go any further. You will be provided with pertinent information only when you ask the appropriate question. For any hands-on procedure, such as auscultation of a blood pressure or breath sounds or taking a pulse, select the appropriate equipment needed (if any) and use the equipment in the manner that it would be used on a patient. I will then give you the relevant clinical data. For example, you must select, place, and begin inflation of the BP cuff before the blood pressure is given to you. I will not answer questions in place of the patient. Therefore, it is imperative that you interact with your patient. Please verbalize to me any signs or symptoms that you find so that I will know you are cognizant of the patient and the patient's clinical appearance. The goal of this station is for you to complete an assessment with emphasis on the use of the SAMPLE and OPQRST history to develop a differential field diagnosis and initiate appropriate treatment.

Scenario

Advise the participants that they are responding to an unknown medical emergency. If the participants are nurses or in-hospital providers, the scenario can be modified to the medical environment—such as the triage nurse brings a patient who complains of "not feeling well" to Medical Room 1. The participant should use the assessment taught in this course.

Initial Impression: 46-year-old female (or male) lying on the couch, clutching her chest

Scene Size-up/General Impression: The scene is safe for entry and exit. No injury is apparent on brief visual exam.

Initial Assessment:

Mental Status—A&O × 3, answering questions.

Airway—Clear and patent at this time.

Breathing—Respirations 28.

Circulation—Radial pulse irregular at 122 bpm.

Disability/Perfusion—Moves all four extremities. Skin cool and clammy.

Status after Initial Assessment: Critical, potentially life threatening.

Possible Differential (Field) Diagnoses: AMI/acute coronary syndrome, pulmonary emboli, dissecting aneurysm.

Initial Management Priorities: High-flow oxygen at 15 lpm via NRM, cardiac monitor, IV access.

Focused History (SAMPLE):

Signs and Symptoms—Pale, cool, clammy skin; clutching her chest.

Allergies—NKA.

Medications—Isosorbide, Lasix.

Past Medical History—Past MI and hypertension, indigestion.

Last Oral Intake—Patient states she had something last night at dinner, but not much, because it hurt to swallow.

Events Preceding—The patient had an endoscopy performed yesterday due to her chronic heart burn and indigestion. When patient woke this morning, she tried to get up, but when she did, she was dizzy and nauseated. She vomited some bloody mucous and now the pain is much worse.

OPQRST:

Onset—It was there when I woke this morning.

Palliation/Provocation—Nothing seems to affect the pain.

Quality—Burning in my chest.

Radiation—It does go into my neck and back.

Severity—On a scale of 1 to 10, it started at a 3–4 and now it is a 7–8.

Time/Duration—Since last night.

Vital Signs:

Respirations—28

Pulse—Radial pulse irregular at 112 bpm (if monitor is placed on patient, it will show sinus tachycardia with occasional PVCs)

Blood Pressure—96/42

Temperature—98.4°F (37°C)

Pulse Oximetry—97%

Blood Glucose Level—106 mg/dl

Focused Physical Exam (Focused Medical Assessment): Nothing significant

Differential/Field Diagnosis: AMI/Acute Coronary Syndrome, pulmonary emboli, aortic dissection, esophageal tear/mediastinitis, esophagitis/reflux

Management:

1) High-flow oxygen at 15 lpm via NRM.

2) IV access.

3) Cardiac monitor—sinus tachycardia with occasional PVCs. (If the participant asks, the pain is not the same as when patient had his [her] last MI.)

4) Rapid transport to appropriate facility.

Critical Actions:

1) Secure airway and ensure highest oxygenation at 15 lpm via NRM; if respiratory failure, then PPV.

2) Maintain hemodynamic stability.

3) Early transport to a facility with surgical capabilities.

Teaching Points

1) There are numerous causes and etiologies of chest pain. Assist the participant in classifying chest pain to body system and causes (e.g., cardiac vs. respiratory, trauma vs. medical) for rule outs.

2) Always follow an organized approach to rule out possible causes.

3) Compare and contrast clinical findings of an AMI to other presentations.

4) Compare and contrast the treatment of an AMI.

5) Discuss the possible differential/field diagnoses

   ▶ *AMI/Acute Coronary Syndrome*—Possible, but ECG is negative at this time, and breath sounds. The patient has a burning-type pain that worsened after vomiting. The pain and the bloody vomit should direct us to an esophageal tear. It would be important to keep this potential diagnosis on the list because this patient could still develop an AMI, so cardiac monitoring should be continued.

   ▶ *Pulmonary emboli*—Possible, but the presentation is more consistent with other diagnoses.

   ▶ *Aortic dissection*—Possible due to pain presentation, but not as likely due to bloody vomit.

   ▶ *Esophageal disruption*—Likely due to reflux history, recent endoscopy, and recent episode of bloody vomit.

Evaluation

1) *Excellent:* The participant's evaluation of the patient followed set format: initial assessment, focused history (SAMPLE, OPQRST) in an efficient manner. The participant displayed a thorough knowledge of the patient's condition, performed the exam and management in an organized manner, identified appropriate differential field diagnoses and demonstrated an excellent overall performance.

2) *Good:* The participant's evaluation of the patient followed set format: initial assessment, focused history (SAMPLE, OPQRST) in an acceptable

manner with only minor deviation. The participant displayed an above-average knowledge of the patient's condition, performed the exam and management of the patient's condition, and demonstrated an above-average performance.

3) *Fair:* The participant's evaluation of the patient deviated from the set format without causing any further injury to the patient. The participant displayed an average or basic knowledge of the patient's condition and performed an adequate exam and management of the patient's condition.

4) *Inadequate:* The participant's evaluation of the patient deviated significantly from the set format, or the participant's actions endangered the patient's life or significantly exacerbated the condition.

▶ CHEST DISCOMFORT: SCENARIO 4

Requirements: One instructor and one patient for every five participants.

Prerequisites: Read Chapter 6, "Chest Discomfort or Pain."

Equipment: One table and chair for the patient to use; jump kit with oxygen supplies (NC, NRM, aerosol mask, PPV device, intubation equipment), stethoscope, BP cuff, cardiac monitor, pulse oximeter (optional but recommended), and medication kit with associated medications.

Instructor: Your role is vital because you must act as the coordinator of the station and also interact in the scenario. Before the participants arrive at the station, please review the scenario with your patient. Spray the patient's arms with a fine mist of cool water to simulate cool and clammy skin. Tint the lip and nail beds blue to simulate cyanosis. Please read the scenario to become familiar with the necessary responses. Do not "coach" the participants along during the testing station; rather, allow them to conduct the exam without interruption or help.

Patient: One female (or male) patient. As the patient, you will be required to play the role of a 56-year-old female (or male) complaining of burning in your chest. You have pneumonia and are having chest pain with a possible myocardial infarction. Please read the scenario and become familiar with the information. You will have a fine mist of water sprayed on you to simulate cool and diaphoretic skin and will have blue moulage applied to your nail beds and lips.

Instructions

Hi, my name is _____, and I will be the examiner for this station. This is a hands-on patient assessment station. You will be given information concerning a patient experiencing a medical crisis. You will have all the necessary equipment you need to manage the patient in this station. Please look over the equipment before we go any further. You will be provided with pertinent information only when you ask the appropriate question. For any hands-on procedure, such as auscultation of a blood pressure or breath sounds or taking a pulse, select the appropriate equipment needed (if any) and use the equipment in the manner that it would be used on a patient. I will then give you the relevant clinical data. For example, you must select, place, and begin inflation of the BP cuff before the blood pressure is given to you. I will not answer questions in place of the patient. Therefore, it is imperative that you interact with your patient. Please verbalize to me any signs or symptoms that you find so that I will know you are cognizant of the patient and the patient's clinical appearance. The goal of this station is for you to complete an assessment with emphasis on use of the SAMPLE and OPQRST history to develop a differential field diagnosis and initiate appropriate treatment.

Scenario

Advise the participants that they are responding to a call of a 56-year-old female (or male) with chest pain. If the participants are nurses or in-hospital providers, the scenario can be modified to the medical environment—such as someone rushes a 56-year-old patient in a wheelchair to your desk. The participant should use the assessment taught in this course.

Initial Impression: 56-year-old female (or male) sitting in a recliner (or wheel-chair). The patient is awake, very anxious, has poor color with cyanosis, and has accessory muscle usage.

Scene Size-up/General Impression: The scene is safe for entry and exit. No injury is apparent on brief visual exam.

Initial Assessment:

Mental Status—Responsive and alert to all commands.

Airway—The patient has a frequent, weak cough.

Breathing—Respirations 26 and very shallow.

Circulation—Radial pulse regular at 98 bpm.

Disability/Perfusion—Moves all four extremities; skin pale, cyanotic, cool, and diaphoretic; distal pulses present.

Status after Initial Assessment: Serious, potentially life threatening.

Possible Differential (Field) Diagnoses: AMI/Acute Coronary Syndrome, aortic dissection, pulmonary embolism, cardiac tamponade, pericarditis, others' options may be presented.

Initial Management Priorities: High-flow oxygen at 15 lpm via NRM, cardiac monitor, IV access

Focused History (SAMPLE):

Signs and Symptoms—Chest pain, respiratory distress, cool and diaphoretic skin.

Allergies—NKA.

Medications—Antibiotic, albuterol, prednisone; all for recent diagnosis of pneumonia.

Past Medical History—Gallstones two years ago.

Last Oral Intake—Patient just finished eating. Cereal.

Events Preceding—Patient states that she had just finished eating and began having chest pain.

OPQRST:

Onset—I haven't been feeling well, chest pain began 20–30 minutes ago. She was resting after having eaten cereal for breakfast.

Palliation/Provocation—Nothing seems to make it better or worse.

Quality—My chest feels tight. I'm hurt from all the coughing, but this is different.

Radiation—In the middle of my chest and back.

Severity—It's a 6 on a 1–10 scale.

Time/Duration—The tightness began before she called. The ache in her chest has been going on for a couple of days.

Vital Signs:

Respirations—26 and shallow, absent breath sounds in left lower lobe.

Pulse—Radial pulse irregular at 98 bpm and bounding.

Blood Pressure—134/96.

Temperature—98.5°F (37°C).

Pulse Oximetry—97%.

Blood Glucose Level—112 mg/dl (6.1 mmol/L).

Focused Physical Exam (Focused Medical Assessment): Patient in respiratory distress. No other findings. Her (his) chest over the sternum area is painful when compressed.

Differential/Field Diagnosis: AMI/Acute Coronary Syndrome, aortic dissection, pulmonary embolism, esophageal tear, cardiac tamponade, pericarditis, pneumonia, costochondritis, pleural effusion.

Management:

1) High-flow oxygen at 15 lpm via NRM.

2) IV access.

3) Cardiac monitor—12 head EKG shows sinus rhythm and ST elevation in V1-2.

4) Nitroglycerin 0.4 mg SL up to three doses for alleviation of pain; hypotension and nitro drip would also be acceptable.

5) Aspirin 160–325 mg orally, preferably chewed.

6) Consider morphine sulfate 2–5 mg IVP if BP does not drop from nitro.

7) Transport to an appropriate facility.

Critical Actions:

1) Secure airway and ensure highest oxygenation at 15 lpm via NRM. Maintain hemodynamic stability.

2) Treat chest pain.

Teaching Points

1) There are numerous causes and etiologies of chest pain. Assist the participant in classifying chest pain to body system and causes (e.g., cardiac vs. respiratory, trauma vs. medical) for rule outs.

2) Always follow an organized approach to rule out possible causes.

3) Compare and contrast clinical findings to other presentations.

4) Review the management of this patient.

5) Discuss the possible differential/field diagnoses.

   ▶ *AMI/Acute Coronary Syndrome*—Likely, because ECG is positive at this time. The patient has pain consistent with an MI. Lung sounds, history, and physical findings suggest pneumonia and costochondritis. Because an AMI is a greater life threat, priority should be on the AMI.

   ▶ *Pulmonary emboli*—Possible, but the presentation is more consistent with other diagnoses.

   ▶ *Aortic dissection*—Possible due to pain presentation, but not as likely due to cardiac changes.

   ▶ *Esophageal disruption*—Possible, the pain and coughing are consistent with esophageal disruption, but no other symptoms. AMI is most likely and should be the focus.

- *Cardiac tamponade*—Not likely, the patient is not hypotensive, no neck vein distention.

- *Pericarditis*—Possible, the chest pain is consistent with pericarditis, the patient has had a recent infection. Not as likely based on ECG.

- *Pneumonia*—Likely due to history, lung sounds, and medications. Not likely the entire problem, but hypoxia could contribute to myocardial hypoxia.

- *Costochondritis*—Possible to due pneumonia, coughing, and chest pain, but not consistent with ECG changes.

Evaluation

1) *Excellent:* The participant's evaluation of the patient followed set format: initial assessment, focused history (SAMPLE, OPQRST) in an efficient manner. The participant displayed a thorough knowledge of the patient's condition, performed the exam and management in an organized manner, identified appropriate differential field diagnoses and demonstrated an excellent overall performance.

2) *Good:* The participant's evaluation of the patient followed set format: initial assessment, focused history (SAMPLE, OPQRST) in an acceptable manner with only minor deviation. The participant displayed an above-average knowledge of the patient's condition, performed the exam and management of the patient's condition, and demonstrated an above-average performance.

3) *Fair:* The participant's evaluation of the patient deviated from the set format without causing any further injury to the patient. The participant displayed an average or basic knowledge of the patient's condition and performed an adequate exam and management of the patient's condition.

4) *Inadequate:* The participant's evaluation of the patient deviated significantly from the set format, or the participant's actions endangered the patient's life or significantly exacerbated the condition.

⊞ ALTERED MENTAL STATUS/SEIZURES AND SEIZURE DISORDERS

▶ ALTERED MENTAL STATUS/SEIZURES AND SEIZURE DISORDERS: SCENARIO 1

Requirements: One instructor and one patient for every five participants.

Prerequisites: Read Chapter 7, "Altered Mental Status" and Chapter 10, "Seizures and Seizure Disorders."

Equipment: One table and chair for the patient to use; jump kit with oxygen supplies (NC, NRM, aerosol mask, PPV device, intubation equipment), stethoscope, BP cuff, cardiac monitor, pulse oximeter, and medication kit with assorted medications.

Instructor: Your role is vital because you must act as the coordinator of the station and also interact in the scenario. Before the participants arrive at the station, please review the scenario with your patient. For moulage, tint the patient's face to simulate pallor.

Patient: One female (or male) patient. As the patient, you will be required to play the role of a 54-year-old suffering from a decreased level of consciousness. Please breathe shallowly and at a rate of approximately 16 breaths per minute You are responsive to verbal and painful stimuli. Please read the scenario to familiarize yourself with the information.

Instructions

Hi, my name is _____, and I will be the instructor for this station. This is a hands-on patient assessment station. You will be given information concerning a patient experiencing a medical crisis. You will have all the necessary equipment you need to manage the patient in this station. Please look over the equipment before we go any further. You will be provided with pertinent information only when you ask the appropriate question. For any hands-on procedure, such as auscultation of a blood pressure or breath sounds or taking a pulse, select the appropriate equipment needed (if any) and use the equipment in the manner that it would be used on a patient. I will then give you the relevant clinical data. For example, you must select, place, and begin inflation of the BP cuff before the blood pressure is given to you. I will not answer questions in place of the patient. Therefore, it is imperative that you interact with your patient. Please verbalize to me any signs or symptoms that you find so that I will know you are cognizant of the patient and the patient's clinical appearance.

Scenario

Advise the participants that they are responding to an unknown medical emergency. If the participants are nurses or in-hospital providers, the scenario can be modified to the medical environment—such as reporting to triage after a shift change and the patient and friend arrive by taxi and pull up to the ED. The participants should use the assessment taught in this course.

Initial Impression: 54-year-old female (or male) in her chair on the aircraft responsive, with complaint of syncope upon standing.

Scene Size-up/General Impression: Airport security, flight attendants, and police are present and escort you to the patient. No evidence of injury noted.

Initial Assessment:

Mental Status—AVPU: Patient is oriented and responds to verbal stimuli.

Airway—Patient able to maintain own airway, but coughs periodically, with greenish sputum.

Breathing—Respirations shallow with periodic coughing.

Circulation—Weak and regular at the radius, with no external bleeding.

Disability/Perfusion—Responsive, but lightheaded when seated fully upright or attempts to stand. Skin warm, pink, and dry.

Status after Initial Assessment: Not immediately life threatening, but unstable.

Possible Differential (Field) Diagnoses: Hypoxia, sepsis, or dehydration secondary to pneumonia/viral syndrome, CNS infection, hypoglycemia, medications, hypovolemia from other cause, vasovagal secondary to anxiety.

Initial Management Priorities: Monitor airway, BSI, cardiac monitor, blood glucose level, oxygen at 15 lpm with NRM, IV therapy, recovery position.

Focused History (SAMPLE):

Signs and Symptoms—Responsive. Skin warm, pink, and dry.

Allergies—None.

Medications—Antiviral medication for 1 day.

Past Medical History—The patient states that no pertinent medical history exists beyond this present illness. **The participants started antiviral medication for an undiagnosed illness, in anticipation the patient was experiencing Avian Flu.**

Last Oral Intake—Water only since flight left Asia.

Events Preceding—Patient states she felt that cough has worsened since leaving Asia 16 hours earlier. Patient is a veterinarian and left work to travel to a conference in North America. Patient prescribed her own antiviral medication just before leaving Asia.

OPQRST:

Onset—Last several days, worse since departure 16 hours ago.

Palliation/Provocation—Nothing is really improving it; standing leads to syncope.

Quality—Severe cough, sore throat, and mild onset of conjunctivitis noted. Some chest discomfort during coughing, and productive cough noted.

Radiation—Pain in chest wall during coughing.

Severity—7 on a 0–10 scale. Describes pleuritic chest pain due to cough.

Time—Last couple of days, more severe in past 16–24 hours.

Vital Signs:

> *Respirations*—16 and shallow, unlabored.

> *Pulse*—Radial pulse 120 bpm and weak at radius.

> *Blood Pressure*—92/70.

> *Temperature*—102.5°F (39.1°C).

> *Pulse Oximetry*—92% with room air, 95% with supplemental O_2.

> *Blood Glucose Level*—92 mg/dl (5.1 mmol/L).

Focused Physical Exam (Focused Medical Assessment): Inspection reveals productive cough, conjunctivitis in right eye, rhonchi noted on auscultation, worse on left lung. Patient appears exhausted and dehydrated. Abdomen tender to palpation due to persistent cough. Purposeful movement in extremities. No neurological deficits noted.

Differential/Field Diagnosis: Syncopal episode prior to arrival at gate. Respiratory infection of unknown etiology. Patient is dehydrated. Syncope is due to respiratory infection, dehydration, and postural hypotension due to extended flight times.

Management:

1) Appropriate body substance isolation, consider quarantine potential (but avoid inciting mass hysteria).

2) Monitoring of airway, management of circulation, and evaluation of O_2 saturation.

3) Supplemental oxygen via simple face mask or non-rebreather mask.

4) IV access—check blood glucose level (BGL)—92 mg/dl (5.1 mmol/L).

5) Fluid bolus.

6) Cardiac monitor—sinus tachycardia without ectopy.

7) Consider bronchodilator medications.

8) Place respiratory protection on patient to prevent spread of possible contagious disease.

9) Patient loses consciousness with postural change.

   a) ABC assessment.

   b) Position patient to facilitate circulatory status.

   c) Re-evaluate fluid resuscitation.

   d) Monitor cardiac rhythmn, and look for other causes of syncope.

   e) Constant re-evaluation of patient condition.

Detailed Physical Exam: En route to appropriate facility if time permits.

Ongoing Assessment: Every 5 minutes en route to appropriate facility.

Critical Actions:

1) Recognize potential for infectious contagion. Apply BSI to self, team members, and patient.

2) Determine appropriate treatment modalities.

Teaching Points

1) There are numerous causes and etiologies of altered mental status.

2) Always follow an organized approach to rule out possible causes.

3) Don't let past medical history lead you to a diagnosis preemptively.

4) Discuss treatment priorities—oxygen administration and protection of airway and fluid resuscitation.

Evaluation

1) *Excellent:* The participant's evaluation of the patient followed set format: initial assessment, focused history (SAMPLE, OPQRST) in an efficient manner. The participant displayed a thorough knowledge of the patient's condition, performed the exam and management in an organized manner, and demonstrated an excellent overall performance.

2) *Good:* The participant's evaluation of the patient followed set format: initial assessment, focused history (SAMPLE, OPQRST) in an acceptable manner with only minor deviation. The participant displayed an above-average knowledge of the patient's condition, performed the exam and management of the patient's condition, and demonstrated an above-average performance.

3) *Fair:* The participant's evaluation of the patient deviated from the set format without causing any further injury to the patient. The participant displayed an average or basic knowledge of the patient's condition and performed an adequate exam and management of the patient's condition.

4) *Inadequate:* The participant's evaluation of the patient deviated significantly from the set format, or the participant's actions endangered the patient's life or significantly exacerbated the condition.

► ALTERED MENTAL STATUS/SEIZURES AND SEIZURE DISORDERS: SCENARIO 2

Requirements: One instructor and one patient for every five participants.

Prerequisites: Read Chapter 7, "Altered Mental Status" and Chapter 10, "Seizures and Seizure Disorders."

Equipment: One table and chair for the patient to use; jump kit with oxygen supplies (NC, NRM, aerosol mask, PPV device, intubation equipment), stethoscope, BP cuff, cardiac monitor, pulse oximeter, and medication kit with assorted medications.

Instructor: Your role is vital because you must act as the coordinator of the station and also interact in the scenario. Before the participants arrive at the station, please review the scenario with your patient. Spray the patient's arms with a fine mist of cool water to simulate cool and clammy skin. For moulage, tint the patient's face with a blue coloring to simulate cyanosis. Have the patient place an artificial blood pill in his mouth. Instruct the patient to break the pill, allowing blood to trickle out of his mouth. You will act as the patient's friend and answer the questions as best as you can.

Patient: One male (or female) patient. As the patient, you will be required to play the role of a 24-year-old male (or female) suffering from a generalized tonic-clonic seizure. Please move your arms and legs, rhythmically interrupted by a short period of "stiffness" of the extremities. You will not respond to any verbal or painful stimuli. Please read the scenario to familiarize yourself with the information.

Instructions

Hi, my name is _____, and I will be the instructor for this station. This is a hands-on patient assessment station. You will be given information concerning a patient experiencing a medical crisis. You will have all the necessary equipment you need to manage the patient in this station. Please look over the equipment before we go any further. You will be provided with pertinent information only when you ask the appropriate question. For any hands-on procedure, such as auscultation of a blood pressure or breath sounds or taking a pulse, select the appropriate equipment needed (if any) and use the equipment in the manner that it would be used on a patient. I will then give you the relevant clinical data. For example, you must select, place, and begin inflation of the BP cuff before the blood pressure is given to you. I will not answer questions in place of the patient. Therefore, it is imperative that you interact with your patient. Please verbalize to me any signs or symptoms that you find so that I will know you are cognizant of the patient and the patient's clinical appearance.

Scenario

Advise the participants that they are responding to a seizure at a local pharmacy. If the participants are nurses or in-hospital providers, the scenario can be modified to the medical environment—such as reporting to triage after a shift change where a patient is lying on the floor apparently having a seizure. The participant should use the assessment taught in this course.

Initial Impression: 24-year-old male (or female) lying supine on the floor flailing around, apparently having a seizure.

Scene Size-up/General Impression: The store manager escorts you to the patient. Store employees have closed the aisle. Police department and EMS have been notified of incident and are responding as well.

Initial Assessment:

Mental Status—AVPU: unresponsive to verbal and painful stimulus. Patient is actively seizing.

Airway—Minimal dried blood in the mouth.

Breathing—Respirations rapid, shallow with wheezes noted.

Circulation—Present, but difficult to assess because of seizure activity; no evidence of injury, no external bleeding.

Disability/Perfusion—Tonic-clonic movement. Skin pale, cool, and dry to touch.

Status after Initial Assessment: Life-threatening, unstable.

Possible Differential (Field) Diagnoses: Pulmonary embolus, epilepsy or undiagnosed seizure disorder, undiagnosed cardiac disorder, severe bronchospasm hypoglycemia with hyposia.

Initial Management Priorities: Suction airway, high-flow positive pressure oxygen with BVM or equivalent if inadequate air exchange. Management is focused on safety of patient initially (protect from injuring self) and maintaining ventilation. Prepare to insert oral or nasal airway and intubate if necessary. Next priority is to stop the seizure (usually with rapid-acting benzodiazepine). When accessible: IV therapy, blood glucose level, pulse oximetry, cardiac monitor, and determine the underlying cause.

Focused History (SAMPLE):

Signs and Symptoms—Unresponsive, peripheral cyanosis, cool and dry skin.

Allergies—No known allergies. Medications—Some sort of puffer for the breathing problem.

Past Medical History—Per friend, the patient has really bad asthma, and it has become worse as the day went on. They were coming to get a refill from the pharmacy as her puffer ran out.

Last Oral Intake—Approximately 3 hours ago.

Events Preceding—The friend states that the patient had been having trouble breathing most of the morning, and the inhaler ran out approximately 1 hour ago. They decided to come to the pharmacy to pick up a new inhaler.

OPQRST:

Onset—It started about 3 minutes ago. Moves all extremities in a tonic-clonic fashion.

Palliation/Provocation—The patient told her friend that this was a "really bad attack."

Quality—Tonic-clonic movement. Radiation—all four extremities.

Severity—Tonic-clonic movement.

Time—Per friend, the "fit" came on after the patient began coughing and wheezing badly until she lost consciousness.

Vital Signs:

Respirations—40 and very shallow (unless PPV was initiated).

Pulse—Irregular radial pulse rapid, 130 bpm, absent at wrist.

Blood Pressure—80/58.

Temperature—99°F (37.1°C).

Pulse Oximetry—Oximeter reads "out of range," poor signal. It will begin to read once O_2 levels have increased, and peripheral perfusion is restored. A reading of 82% would be found if the SpO_2 monitor probes are attached to a "central location" like the ear lobe.

Focused Physical Exam (Focused Medical Assessment): Patient continues to have tonic-clonic movement that diminishes with PPV, blood from mouth indicates possible tongue laceration. Lung sounds reveal silence in the bases bilaterally, with fine wheezes noted with PPV in the apices bilaterally.

Differential/Field Diagnoses: Acute, generalized seizure related to hypoxia.

Management:

1) Suction of oral pharynx, if possible.

2) Insertion of OPA and/or NPA.

3) PPV with BVM, high-flow O_2 administration.

4) IV access—check BGL—88 mg/dl (4.8 mmol/L).

5) Cardiac monitor, when obtainable—sinus tachycardia with multifocal PVCs.

6) Note: If patient is still actively seizing, priority would be to give benzo for seizure. Then if bronchospasm noted, give bronchodilators administered via BVM. IV administration of Epinephrine should be considered if bronchospasm severe or if patient thought to have anaphylaxis; when time permits, solumedrol or solucortef; consider fluid bolus.

Detailed Physical Exam: En route to appropriate facility if time permits.

Ongoing Assessment: Every 5 minutes while en route to the receiving facility.

Critical Actions:

1) Suction and secure airway, insert OPA or NPA.

2) Stop the seizure activity.

Teaching Points

1) There are numerous causes and etiologies of seizures.

2) Always follow an organized approach to rule out possible causes.

3) Don't let past medical history lead you to a diagnosis preemptively.

4) Discuss treatment priorities—suction and protect airway and provide O_2. Early intubation is not always warranted. Highest priority is to stop the seizure activity, then assess for potential causes of the seizure and ongoing problems that need to be treated such as hypoxia.

5) Discuss the limitations of pulse oximeters in the presence of poor peripheral perfusion. Encourage discussion of participant's devices, and consider probe attachment to the earlobe as a more central location to evaluate perfusion.

6) Discuss how bronchodilators can be administered (PPV) if IV access is not possible due to seizure activity.

Evaluation

1) *Excellent:* The participant's evaluation of the patient followed set format: initial assessment, focused history (SAMPLE, OPQRST) in an efficient manner. The participant displayed a thorough knowledge of the patient's condition, performed the exam and management in an organized manner, and demonstrated an excellent overall performance.

2) *Good:* The participant's evaluation of the patient followed set format: initial assessment, focused history (SAMPLE, OPQRST) in an acceptable manner with only minor deviation. The participant displayed an above-average knowledge of the patient's condition, performed the exam and management of the patient's condition, and demonstrated an above-average performance.

3) *Fair:* The participant's evaluation of the patient deviated from the set format without causing any further injury to the patient. The participant displayed an average or basic knowledge of the patient's condition and performed an adequate exam and management of the patient's condition.

4) *Inadequate:* The participant's evaluation of the patient deviated significantly from the set format, or the participant's actions endangered the patient's life or significantly exacerbated the condition.

▶ ALTERED MENTAL STATUS/SEIZURES AND SEIZURE DISORDERS: SCENARIO 3

Requirements: One instructor and one patient for every five participants.

Prerequisites: Read Chapter 7, "Altered Mental Status" and Chapter 10, "Seizures and Seizure Disorders."

Equipment: One table and chair for the patient to use; jump kit with oxygen supplies (NC, NRM, aerosol mask, PPV device, intubation equipment), stethoscope, BP cuff, cardiac monitor, pulse oximeter, and medication kit with assorted medications.

Instructor: Your role is vital because you must act as the coordinator of the station and also interact in the scenario. Before the participant arrives at the station, please review the scenario with your patient. Spray the patient's arms with a fine mist of cool water to simulate cool and clammy skin. For moulage, tint the patient's face with a blue coloring to simulate cyanosis.

Patient: One female (or male) patient. As the patient, you will be required to play the role of a 22-year-old female suffering from a decreased level of consciousness. You will be unresponsive to verbal stimuli and moan when deep, painful stimuli is performed. Place a small amount of liquid in your mouth to simulate gurgling respirations. Please read the scenario to familiarize yourself with the information.

Instructions

Hi, my name is _____, and I will be the instructor for this station. This is a hands-on patient assessment station. You will be given information concerning a patient experiencing a medical crisis. You will have all the necessary equipment you need to manage the patient in this station. Please look over the equipment before we go any further. You will be provided with pertinent information only when you ask the appropriate question. For any hands-on procedure, such as auscultation of a blood pressure or breath sounds or taking a pulse, select the appropriate equipment needed (if any) and use the equipment in the manner that it would be used on a patient. I will then give you the relevant clinical data. For example, you must select, place, and begin inflation of the BP cuff before the blood pressure is given to you. I will not answer questions in place of the patient. Therefore, it is imperative that you interact with your patient. Please verbalize to me any signs or symptoms that you find so that I will know you are cognizant of the patient and the patient's clinical appearance.

Scenario

Advise the participants that they are responding to a possible overdose. On the scene is a friend who found the patient lying on the bathroom floor with the medicine cabinet open. If the participants are nurses or in-hospital providers, the scenario can be modified to the medical environment—such as reporting to triage after a shift change where a hysterical friend drags the patient into the ED. The participant should use the assessment taught in this course.

Initial Impression: 24-year-old female (or male) lying supine on the floor, unresponsive, with gurgling respirations.

Scene Size-up/General Impression: There is easy access in and out of the residence. Patient's friend escorts you to patient lying on bathroom floor.

Initial Assessment:

Mental Status—AVPU: unresponsive to verbal commands, moans to deep painful stimuli.

Airway—Small amount of saliva in oral pharynx.

Breathing—Respirations very shallow, unlabored.

Circulation—Radial pulse weak and thready, irregular; there is no evidence of injury or bleeding.

Disability/Perfusion—Moans to painful stimuli. Skin pale, cool, and diaphoretic.

Status after Initial Assessment: Life-threatening, unstable.

Possible Differential (Field) Diagnoses: Head trauma related to fall, CVA, non-traumatic cerebral hemorrhage, seizure disorder, overdose due to alcohol, hypoglycemia, hypoxia.

Initial Management Priorities: Airway maintenance with nasal or oral airway device, oxygen at 15 lpm via NRM, pulse oximetry, IV therapy, monitor, recovery position, prepare to intubate.

Focused History (SAMPLE):

Signs and Symptoms—Unresponsive, peripheral cyanosis, cool and clammy skin.

Allergies—Friend doesn't know.

Medications—In the medicine cabinet are OTC analgesic and sinus medications along with TB syringes and alcohol pads.

Past Medical History—Per friend, the patient is very reclusive and is unaware of any.

Last Oral Intake—Per friend, this morning at breakfast.

Events Preceding—The friend states that they had met this morning for breakfast at the mall. The patient looked ill and wasn't feeling well. Consequently, she didn't eat anything and went home to "sleep off her headache."

OPQRST:

Onset—Unknown

Palliation/Provocation—Unknown

Quality—Unknown

Radiation—Unknown

Severity—Unknown

Time—Unknown

Vital Signs:

Respirations—8 and shallow (unless PPV was initiated)

Pulse—Radial pulse weak and thready at 128 bpm

Blood Pressure—98/66

Temperature—98.2°F (36.8°C)

Pulse Oximetry—88% on room air, increases to 90% with supplemental O_2, and 95% with PPV O_2

Blood Glucose Level—48 mg/dl (2.6 mmol/L)

Focused Physical Exam (Focused Medical Assessment): Patient remains responsive only to deep painful stimuli; pupils equal and reactive to light, but a little slow to react. No bruising or injury noted. No medical alert identification found.

Differential/Field Diagnosis: Unresponsive with hypoglycemic episode.

Management:
1) C-spine control
2) Suction of oral pharynx, if possible
3) Insertion of OPA and/or NPA
4) PPV ventilation with supplemental oxygen
5) IV access—check BGL—48 mg/dl
6) Dextrose (D_{50}) 25 grams slow IVP—glucagon 1 mg IM if IV unobtainable
7) Cardiac monitor—sinus tachycardia with occasional PACs

Detailed Physical Exam: En route to appropriate facility if time permits.

Ongoing Assessment: Every 5 minutes while en route to the receiving facility.

Critical Actions:
1) Suction and secure airway, insert OPA or NPA.
2) Check BGL and pupils to determine possible causes.

Teaching Points

1) There are numerous causes and etiologies of an unknown unresponsive.

2) Always follow an organized approach to rule out possible causes.

3) Don't let scene clues lead you to a diagnosis preemptively. (The patient could have been trying to get some sugar candies out of the medicine cabinet when she collapsed.)

4) Discuss treatment priorities—suction and protect airway. Early intubation is not always warranted. Highest priority is to provide glucose to the body.

Evaluation

1) *Excellent:* The participant's evaluation of the patient followed set format: initial assessment, focused history (SAMPLE, OPQRST) in an efficient manner. The participant displayed a thorough knowledge of the patient's condition, performed the exam and management in an organized manner, and demonstrated an excellent overall performance.

2) *Good:* The participant's evaluation of the patient followed set format: initial assessment, focused history (SAMPLE, OPQRST) in an acceptable manner with only minor deviation. The participant displayed an above-average knowledge of the patient's condition, performed the exam and management of the patient's condition, and demonstrated an above-average performance.

3) *Fair:* The participant's evaluation of the patient deviated from the set format without causing any further injury to the patient. The participant displayed an average or basic knowledge of the patient's condition and performed an adequate exam and management of the patient's condition.

4) *Inadequate:* The participant's evaluation of the patient deviated significantly from the set format, or the participant's actions endangered the patient's life or significantly exacerbated the condition.

▶ ALTERED MENTAL STATUS/SEIZURES AND SEIZURE DISORDERS: SCENARIO 4

Requirements: One instructor and one patient for every five participants.

Prerequisites: Read Chapter 7, "Altered Mental Status" and Chapter 10, "Seizures and Seizure Disorders."

Equipment: One table and chair for the patient to use; jump kit with oxygen supplies (NC, NRM, aerosol mask, PPV device, intubation equipment), stethoscope, BP cuff, cardiac monitor, pulse oximeter, and medication kit with assorted medications.

Instructor: Your role is vital because you must act as the coordinator of the station and also interact in the scenario. Before the participants arrive at the station, please review the scenario with your patient. Spray the patient's arms with a fine mist of cool water to simulate cool and clammy skin. You will act as the patient's spouse and answer all questions.

Patient: One male (or female) patient. As the patient, you will be required to play the role of a 32-year-old male (or female) suffering from an acute decreased level of consciousness. You will be unresponsive to verbal stimuli and moan when deep painful stimuli is performed. Please breathe at a very fast and shallow rate, approximately 40 times per minute. Please read the scenario to familiarize yourself with the information.

Instructions

Hi, my name is _____, and I will be the instructor for this station. This is a hands-on patient assessment station. You will be given information concerning a patient experiencing a medical crisis. You will have all the necessary equipment you need to manage the patient in this station. Please look over the equipment before we go any further. You will be provided with pertinent information only when you ask the appropriate question. For any hands-on procedure, such as auscultation of a blood pressure or breath sounds or taking a pulse, select the appropriate equipment needed (if any) and use the equipment in the manner that it would be used on a patient. I will then give you the relevant clinical data. For example, you must select, place, and begin inflation of the BP cuff before the blood pressure is given to you. I will not answer questions in place of the patient. Therefore, it is imperative that you interact with your patient. Please verbalize to me any signs or symptoms that you find so that I will know you are cognizant of the patient and the patient's clinical appearance.

Scenario

Advise the participants that they are responding to a "man down" call. They arrive on scene to find the patient on the floor in the bedroom. If the participants are nurses or in-hospital providers, the scenario can be modified to the medical environment—such as reporting to triage after a shift change where an anxious wife has run into the waiting room asking for help to get her spouse out of the car. The participant should use the assessment taught in this course.

Initial Impression: 32-year-old male (or female) lying supine on the floor.

Scene Size-up/General Impression: Neighbor lets you access the home from the front door. There is easy access in and out of the residence. There are no animals or appearance of violence.

Initial Assessment:

Mental Status—AVPU: unresponsive to verbal commands, moans to deep painful stimuli; no injury apparent.

Airway—Clear and patent at this time.

Breathing—Respirations 40, irregular pattern noted.

Circulation—Radial pulse bounding at 50 bpm, no external bleeding present.

Disability/Perfusion—Distal pulses strong and bounding. Skin flushed, dry, and warm.

Status after Initial Assessment: Life-threatening, unstable.

Possible Differential (Field) Diagnoses: Diabetes, overdose or heat-related syncope, head trauma, cerebral hemorrhage, CVA, sepsis.

Initial Management Priorities: Airway maintenance with oral or nasal airway, intubation recommended. High flow O_2 via bag-valve-mask. Pulse oximetry, cardiac monitor, IV therapy, blood glucose level, suction if necessary.

Focused History (SAMPLE):

Signs and Symptoms—Unresponsive with pathological respiratory pattern noted.

Allergies—Spouse states none.

Medications—Adalat.

Past Medical History—Significant for hypertension.

Last Oral Intake—This morning at breakfast.

Events Preceding—The spouse states that they had just finished having sexual intercourse when the patient got out of bed to use the bathroom. He complained of a "killer headache, the worst he ever had" and then suddenly collapsed on the floor.

OPQRST:

Onset—Rapid.

Palliation/Provocation—Unknown.

Quality—Unknown.

Radiation—Spouse states that the patient had said the pain was just in his head.

Severity—"Killer headache, the worst of his life."

Time—Approximately 20 minutes ago.

Vital Signs:

Respirations—40 and very shallow and irregular (unless PPV was initiated).

Pulse—Radial pulse strong, regular & bounding at 50 bpm.

Blood Pressure—214/168.

Temperature—101°F (38.3°C).

Pulse Oximetry—90% without 02, 95% with 02 via PPV.

Blood Glucose Level—112 mg/dl (6.2 mmol/L).

Focused Physical Exam (Focused Medical Assessment): Patient remains responsive only to deep painful stimuli; right pupil is dilated and non-reactive. No signs of injury present.

Differential/Field Diagnosis: Possible cerebral (intracranial) bleeding.

Management:

1) Insertion of OPA and/or NPA

2) PPV ventilation with supplemental oxygen

3) IV access

4) Cardiac monitor—sinus tachycardia with no ectopy

5) Endotracheal intubation via RSI

   a) Defasciculating agent—vecuronium 0.01 mg/kg IVP

   b) Sedative—midazolam 0.05–0.1 mg/kg IVP, diazepam 0.2 mg/kg IVP, fentanyl 3–5 µg/kg, or any of the other sedatives

   c) Cricoid pressure

   d) Succinylcholine 1.5 mg/kg IVP

   e) Intubation

   f) Confirmation

6) Positive pressure ventilation to help decrease intracranial pressure; hyperventilate only if signs of herniation

7) Rapid transport to appropriate facility

Detailed Physical Exam: En route to appropriate facility if time permits.

Ongoing Assessment: En route to the receiving facility every 5 minutes.

Critical Actions:

1) PPV with supplemental oxygen.

2) Endotracheal intubation with RSI to secure the airway and provide ventilation.

3) Do not treat with hypertonic or dextrose solutions.

4) DO NOT TREAT THE ELEVATED BLOOD PRESSURE (until CAT scan demonstrates bleeding).

Teaching Points

1) There are numerous causes and etiologies of an unknown unresponsive.

2) Always follow an organized approach to rule out possible causes.

3) Don't let scene clues lead you to a diagnosis preemptively. (As humorous as the scene may have initially appeared, the outcome was deadly.)

4) Discuss treatment priorities—PPV with supplemental oxygen and RSI.

5) Discuss the effects of dextrose and hypertonic solutions.

6) Discuss the effects of lowering the blood pressure.

Evaluation

1) *Excellent:* The participant's evaluation of the patient followed set format: initial assessment, focused history (SAMPLE, OPQRST) in an efficient manner. The participant displayed a thorough knowledge of the patient's condition, performed the exam and management in an organized manner, and demonstrated an excellent overall performance.

2) *Good:* The participant's evaluation of the patient followed set format: initial assessment, focused history (SAMPLE, OPQRST) in an acceptable manner with only minor deviation. The participant displayed an above-average knowledge of the patient's condition, performed the exam and management of the patient's condition, and demonstrated an above-average performance.

3) *Fair:* The participant's evaluation of the patient deviated from the set format without causing any further injury to the patient. The participant displayed an average or basic knowledge of the patient's condition and performed an adequate exam and management of the patient's condition.

4) *Inadequate:* The participant's evaluation of the patient deviated significantly from the set format, or the participant's actions endangered the patient's life or significantly exacerbated the condition.

⊞ ACUTE ABDOMINAL PAIN/GI BLEEDING

▶ ACUTE ABDOMINAL PAIN/GI BLEEDING: SCENARIO 1

Requirements: One instructor and one patient for every five participants.

Prerequisites: Read Chapter 8, "Acute Abdominal Pain"; Chapter 9, "Gastrointestinal Bleeding"; and Chapter 12, "Headache, Nausea, and Vomiting."

Equipment: One table and chair for the patient to use; jump kit with oxygen supplies (NC, NRM, aerosol mask, PPV device, intubation equipment), stethoscope, BP cuff, cardiac monitor, pulse oximeter (optional but encouraged), and medication kit with associated medications.

Instructor: Your role is vital because you must act as the coordinator of the station and also interact in the scenario. Before the participants arrive at the station, please review the scenario with your patient. For moulage, tint the patient's face and arms with a white coloring to simulate pale skin. Please read the scenario to become familiar with the necessary responses. Encourage the participant to use the assessment format described during the assessment station with an emphasis on the SAMPLE and OPQRST history, and differential field diagnosis allow them to conduct the exam without interruption or help.

Patient: One female (or male) patient. As the patient, you will be required to play the role of a 68-year-old female (or male) suffering from acute abdominal pain. You are awake and alert and can answer all questions. The pain started right after breakfast this morning. The pain is a "burning pain" in the upper-left quadrant abdominal area. Your medical history includes angina, for which you take an aspirin a day and nitroglycerin when needed. You also take glucosamine, gingko, ginseng, and vitamin E, and Motrin on occasion for your arthritis. You are lying supine on the couch, with your legs flexed. Please read the scenario to become familiar with the information.

Instructions

Hi, my name is _____, and I will be the coordinator for this station. This is a hands-on patient assessment station. You will be given information concerning a patient experiencing a medical crisis. You will have all the necessary equipment you need to manage the patient in this station. Please look over the equipment before we go any further. You will be provided with pertinent information only when you ask the appropriate question. For any hands-on procedure, such as auscultation of a blood pressure or breath sounds or taking a pulse, select the appropriate equipment needed (if any) and use the equipment in the manner that it would be used on a patient. I will then give you the relevant clinical data. For example, you must select, place, and begin inflation of the BP cuff before the blood pressure is given to you. I will not answer questions in place of the patient. Therefore, it is imperative that you interact with your patient. Please verbalize to me any signs or symptoms that you find so that I will know you are cognizant of the patient and the patient's clinical appearance. The goal of this station is for you to complete an assessment with emphasis on use of the SAMPLE and OPQRST history to develop a differential field diagnosis and initiate appropriate treatment.

Scenario

Advise the participants that they are responding to a call of dizziness and nausea. If the participants are nurses or in-hospital providers, the scenario can be modified to the medical environment—such as a van has pulled up and the spouse has come into the ED to get you. The participant should use the assessment taught in this course.

Initial Impression: 68-year-old female (or male) lying supine with knees slightly flexed on the couch, complaining of dizziness and nausea.

Scene Size-up/General Impression: The scene is safe for entry and exit. No injury is apparent on brief visual exam. Family escorts you to the patient.

Initial Assessment:

Mental Status—Responsive, A&O × 3, GCS 15.

Airway—Open and patent.

Breathing—Respirations 18 and regular, breath sounds equal and clear bilateral.

Circulation—Radial pulse 98 and regular, skin cool and moist.

Disability/Perfusion—Obeys all commands, skin pale and cool, pulses present, but weak.

Status after Initial Assessment: Serious, no immediate intervention needed at this time.

Possible Differential (Field) Diagnoses: Flu, AMI, cardiac dysrhythmia, GI bleeding, gastric or duodenal ulcer, kidney stone or infection, pneumonia, pancreatitis.

Initial Management Priorities: Oxygen at 15 lpm via NRM, cardiac monitor, IV access.

Focused History (SAMPLE):

Signs and Symptoms—Dizziness and nausea, some burning abdominal pain

Allergies—NKA

Medications—Aspirin, nitroglycerin, vitamin E, glucosamine, ginkgo, ginseng

Past Medical History—Angina, arthritis

Last Oral Intake—Breakfast, but didn't eat much because she wasn't feeling well, hasn't felt like eating much for the last few days.

Events Preceding—This morning the patient didn't feel well and had some dizziness, nausea, and vague burning abdominal pain.

OPQRST:

Onset—It started this morning, but she hasn't been feeling well for a while.

Palliation/Provocation—When I lie down, I'm not as dizzy.

Quality—Cramping type of pain.

Radiation—No radiation.

Severity—On a scale of 1 to 10, it's a 6.

Time/Duration—Since this morning. Several hours.

Vital Signs:

Respirations—18 and regular.

Pulse—Radial pulse 98 bpm and regular.

Blood Pressure—110/78, positive orthostatics (tilt test) if evaluated. Heart increases to 120, BP drops to 90/66.

Temperature—98.2°F (36.8°C).

Pulse Oximetry—97%.

Blood Glucose Level—120 mg/dl (6.6 mmol/L).

Focused Physical Exam (Focused Medical Assessment): Rapid head-to-toe, patient's upper left abdomen is tender to palpation. She has weak distal (dorsal pedis) pulses. No vomiting. Dark (blackish color) loose stools for a few days.

Differential/Field Diagnosis: Gastroenteritis, AMI, cardiac dysrhythmia, GI bleeding, distended spleen, gastric or duodenal ulcer, kidney stone or infection, left lung pneumonia, others as appropriate.

Management:

1) High-flow oxygen at 15 lpm via NRM.

2) Do not have the patient stand or walk to cot. Place patient in position of comfort.

3) Rapid transport to an appropriate level facility.

4) Establish two large-bore IVs of NS or LR. Fluid bolus would be acceptable.

5) Cardiac monitor—normal sinus rhythm with no ectopy, 12 lead ECG negative.

6) Continue to monitor respiratory and cardiovascular status. Maintain position of comfort.

Critical Actions:

1) Use assessment clues to come to the field diagnosis.

2) Recognize the potential for an unstable situation.

3) Transport gently and rapidly.

Teaching Points

1) There are numerous causes and etiologies of abdominal pain. Assist the participants in classifying abdominal pain to body system and causes (e.g., cardiovascular vs. gastrointestinal, trauma vs. medical) for rule outs.

2) Always follow an organized approach to rule out possible causes.

3) Don't let past medical history lead you to a diagnosis preemptively.

4) Discuss the need to evaluate for medication use both prescribed and supplement.

5) Discuss the need for early and timely transport due to positive orthostatics.

6) Discuss the possible differential/field diagnoses

   ▶ Gastroenteritis—Possible, but keep other more life-threatening diagnoses on the list. The possibility of GI bleeding is a much greater concern.

   ▶ AMI—Possible due to history, but history indicates another cause. It would be important to keep this potential diagnosis on the list, due to the stress the patient is experiencing. Even though the ECG is negative, damage may still be a potential, so cardiac monitoring should be continued.

   ▶ Cardiac dysrhythmia—Possible due to dizziness, but not likely based on history and current rhythm.

   ▶ GI bleeding, gastric or duodenal Ulcer—Very likely due to medication history; ASA and motrin (ibuprofen) are associated with ulcers. The herbal medications the patient is taking have anticoagulant actions and may contribute to GI bleeding. Tarry stools and positive orthostatic pressures also suggest a GI bleed. Burning pain is commonly associated with ulcers. The upper left quadrant pain and pain relief with flexed knees may signal a perforated ulcer and possible peritonitis.

   ▶ Kidney stone or infection—Possible, but not likely due to pain description and patient presentation.

   ▶ Left lung pneumonia—Not likely due to clear lungs sounds and no recent respiratory involvement.

Evaluation

1) *Excellent:* The participant's evaluation of the patient followed set format: initial assessment, focused history (SAMPLE, OPQRST) in an efficient manner. The participant displayed a thorough knowledge of the patient's condition, performed the exam and management in an organized manner identified appropriate differential field diagnoses, and demonstrated an excellent overall performance.

2) *Good:* The participant's evaluation of the patient followed set format: initial assessment, focused history (SAMPLE, OPQRST) in an acceptable manner with only minor deviation. The participant displayed above-average knowledge of the patient's condition, performed the exam and management of the patient's condition, and demonstrated an above-average performance.

3) *Fair:* The participant's evaluation of the patient deviated from the set format without causing any further injury to the patient. The participant displayed an average or basic knowledge of the patient's condition and performed an adequate exam and management of the patient's condition.

4) *Inadequate:* The participant's evaluation of the patient deviated significantly from the set format, or the participant's actions endangered the patient's life or significantly exacerbated the condition.

► ACUTE ABDOMINAL PAIN/GI BLEEDING: SCENARIO 2

Requirements: One instructor and one patient for every five participants.

Prerequisites: Read Chapter 8, "Acute Abdominal Pain"; Chapter 9, "Gastrointestinal Bleeding"; and Chapter 12, "Headache, Nausea, and Vomiting."

Equipment: One table and chair for the patient to use; jump kit with oxygen supplies (NC, NRM, aerosol mask, PPV device, intubation equipment), stethoscope, BP cuff, cardiac monitor, pulse oximeter (optional but encouraged), and medication kit with associated medications.

Instructor: Your role is vital because you must act as the coordinator of the station and also interact in the scenario. Before the participants arrive at the station, please review the scenario with your patient. For moulage, tint the patient's face with white coloring to simulate pale skin. Encourage the participants to use the assessment format described during the assessment station with an emphasis on the SAMPLE and OPQRST history and differential field diagnoses. Allow them to conduct the exam with minimal interruption or help.

Patient: One male (or female) patient. As the patient, you will be required to play the role of a 17-year-old male (or female) suffering from abdominal pain with vomiting. You will be awake and alert. Please read the scenario to become familiar with the information.

Instructions

Hi, my name is _____, and I will be the coordinator for this station. This is a hands-on patient assessment station. You will be given information concerning a patient experiencing a medical crisis. You will have all the necessary equipment you need to manage the patient in this station. Please look over the equipment before we go any further. You will be provided with pertinent information only when you ask the appropriate question. For any hands-on procedure, such as auscultation of a blood pressure or breath sounds or taking a pulse, select the appropriate equipment needed (if any) and use the equipment in the manner that it would be used on a patient. I will then give you the relevant clinical data. For example, you must select, place, and begin inflation of the BP cuff before the blood pressure is given to you. I will not answer questions in place of the patient. Therefore, it is imperative that you interact with your patient. Please verbalize to me any signs or symptoms that you find so that I will know you are cognizant of the patient and the patient's clinical appearance. The goal of this station is for you to complete an assessment with emphasis on the use of the SAMPLE and OPQRST history to develop a differential field diagnosis and initiate appropriate treatment.

Scenario

Advise the participants that they are responding to an abdominal pain call. If the participants are nurses or in-hospital providers, the scenario can be modified to the medical environment—such as the patient walked into the ED and is sitting in the triage seat. The participant should use the assessment taught in this course.

Initial Impression: 17-year-old male (or female) sitting in a chair, doubled over complaining of a pain in his stomach.

Scene Size-up/General Impression: The scene is safe for entry and exit. No injury is apparent on brief visual exam.

Initial Assessment:

Mental Status—Responsive to all commands.

Airway—Clear at this moment, but the patient does have bouts of nausea.

Breathing—Respirations 20 and very shallow.

Circulation—Radial pulse rapid and strong.

Disability/Perfusion—Moves all four extremities, skin pale and dry.

Status after Initial Assessment: No immediate life threat.

Possible Differential (Field) Diagnoses: Appendicitis, ectopic pregnancy or ruptured ovarian cyst if female, incarcerated hernia, regional ileitis, kidney stone, bowel obstruction, pelvic inflammatory disease, pancreatitis, cholecystitis, peptic ulcer.

Initial Management Priorities: Oxygen, cardiac monitor, IV access, position of comfort.

Focused History (SAMPLE):

Signs and Symptoms—Responsive, pale skin.

Allergies—NKA.

Medications—None.

Past Medical History—None, had the flu with nausea and vomiting last week. Sexually active. If female, her last menstrual period was 6 weeks ago. She could possibly be pregnant.

Last Oral Intake—Ate some crackers a few hours ago, but wasn't feeling well.

Events Preceding—The pain started 4 hours ago and has been getting progressively worse.

OPQRST:

Onset—It started slowly about 4 hours ago.

Palliation/Provocation—It's worse when I move.

Quality—It comes and goes. The pain is becoming more constant.

Radiation—My whole stomach hurts. Now it is worse here and points to lower-right quadrant.

Severity—It's a lot worse when I move. 8 on a 0–10 scale.

Time/Duration—It got worse approximately 4 hours ago.

Vital Signs:

Respirations—20 and shallow.

Pulse—Radial pulse rapid and strong. Rate 92, normal sinus rhythm.

Blood Pressure—128/86, orthostatics (tilt test) negative if done. Heart rate does increase slightly and patient complains of severe pain.

Temperature—98.8°F (37°C).

Pulse Oximetry—99%.

Blood Glucose Level—107 mg/dl.

Focused Physical Exam (Focused Medical Assessment): Patient appears to have increasing pain; nausea and pain is worse on palpation if patient is moved or bumped, pain is severe in lower-right quadrant. No change in stools or urine. No vaginal discharge if female. Guarding on palpation, but no distention or masses noted.

Differential/Field Diagnosis: Appendicitis, ectopic pregnancy or ovarian cyst if female, incarcerated hernia, acute colitis regional ileitis, kidney stone, bowel obstruction, pelvic inflammatory disease.

Management:

1) Supplemental oxygen as needed. Nasal cannula is acceptable.

2) IV access, two large bores (14–16 gauge) with 250–500 cc fluid bolus is acceptable, or titrate to blood pressure.

3) Cardiac monitor.

4) Transport in position of comfort.

5) Pain management as indicated.

Critical Actions:

1) Monitor airway and apply supplemental oxygen as indicated.

2) Monitor hemodynamic stability and administer fluids as indicated.

Teaching Points

1) There are numerous causes and etiologies of abdominal pain. Assist the participants in classifying abdominal pain to body system and causes (e.g., cardiovascular vs. gastrointestinal, trauma vs. medical) for rule outs.

2) Always follow an organized approach to rule out possible causes.

3) Correlate past medical history with possible diagnoses.

4) Treatment priorities are to maintain oxygenation and hemodynamic stability. Consider pain management as indicated.

5) Discuss the possible differential/field diagnoses

▶ Appendicitis—Likely due to pain location and localization of pain to the right-lower quadrant. The pain is worsened by movement or light palpation (peritoneal signs) (positive Rovsing sign), or referred tenderness (i.e., push on lower-left quadrant causes pain in lower-right quadrant). Nausea, vomiting, and anorexia are also consistent with appendicitis.

▶ Ectopic pregnancy or ovarian cyst (if female)—Possible due to history. Ectopic pregnancy pain is usually colicky. Monitor for radiation of pain to the shoulder. It would be important to keep this potential diagnosis on the list, due to the potential for rupture and bleeding, so frequent re-evaluation of hemodynamic status is indicated.

- Incarcerated hernia—Possible due to abdominal pain and vomiting. Pain is usually more severe and usually begins as crampy, then progresses to poorly localized pain. No mass noted. More common in males than females.

- Acute colitis or regional ileitis (Crohn's disease)—Possible, but commonly associated with bouts of diarrhea. No past history of Crohn's disease.

- Kidney stone or infection—Possible, but not likely due to pain description and patient presentation.

- Bowel obstruction—Possible, but not as likely. Pain is usually crampy and progresses to a poorly localized pain. Abdominal distention is usually present as well.

- Pelvic Inflammatory Disease—Possible due to history, but not as likely due to pain presentation. Tubo-ovarian abscess still a concern.

Evaluation

1) *Excellent:* The participant's evaluation of the patient followed set format: initial assessment, focused history (SAMPLE, OPQRST) in an efficient manner. The participant displayed a thorough knowledge of the patient's condition, performed the exam and management in an organized manner, identified appropriate differential field diagnoses, and demonstrated an excellent overall performance.

2) *Good:* The participant's evaluation of the patient followed set format: initial assessment, focused history (SAMPLE, OPQRST) in an acceptable manner with only minor deviation. The participant displayed an above-average knowledge of the patient's condition, performed the exam and management of the patient's condition, and demonstrated an above-average performance.

3) *Fair:* The participant's evaluation of the patient deviated from the set format without causing any further injury to the patient. The participant displayed an average or basic knowledge of the patient's condition and performed an adequate exam and management of the patient's condition.

4) *Inadequate:* The participant's evaluation of the patient deviated significantly from the set format, or the participant's actions endangered the patient's life or significantly exacerbated the condition.

▶ ACUTE ABDOMINAL PAIN/GI BLEEDING: SCENARIO 3

Requirements: One instructor and one patient for every five participants.

Prerequisites: Read Chapter 8, "Acute Abdominal Pain"; Chapter 9, "Gastrointestinal Bleeding"; and Chapter 12, "Headache, Nausea, and Vomiting."

Equipment: One table and chair for the patient to use; jump kit with oxygen supplies (NC, NRM, aerosol mask, PPV device, intubation equipment), stethoscope, BP cuff, cardiac monitor, pulse oximeter (optional but encouraged), and medication kit with associated medications.

Instructor: Your role is vital because you must act as the coordinator of the station and also interact in the scenario. Before the participants arrive at the station, please review the scenario with your patient. Please read the scenario to become familiar with the necessary responses. Do not "coach" the participants along during the testing station; rather, allow them to conduct the exam without interruption or help.

Patient: One female patient. As the patient, you will be required to play the role of a 36-year-old female complaining of acute abdominal pain. You will be awake and alert and cooperative. Please read the scenario to become familiar with the information.

Instructions

Hi, my name is _____, and I will be the examiner for this station. This is a hands-on patient assessment station. You will be given information concerning a patient experiencing a medical crisis. You will have all the necessary equipment you need to manage the patient in this station. Please look over the equipment before we go any further. You will be provided with pertinent information only when you ask the appropriate question. For any hands-on procedure, such as auscultation of a blood pressure or breath sounds or taking a pulse, select the appropriate equipment needed (if any) and use the equipment in the manner that it would be used on a patient. I will then give you the relevant clinical data. For example, you must select, place, and begin inflation of the BP cuff before the blood pressure is given to you. I will not answer questions in place of the patient. Therefore, it is imperative that you interact with your patient. Please verbalize to me any signs or symptoms that you find so that I will know you are cognizant of the patient and the patient's clinical appearance. The goal of this station is for you to complete an assessment with emphasis on use of the SAMPLE and OPQRST history to develop a differential field diagnosis and initiate appropriate treatment.

Scenario

Advise the participants that they are responding to the home of a 36-year-old female with abdominal pain. If the participants are nurses or in-hospital providers, the scenario can be modified to the medical environment—such as a new patient with abdominal pain is in Medical Room 5. The participant should use the assessment taught in this course.

Initial Impression: 36-year-old female lying on the couch on her side with her knees drawn up.

Scene Size-up/General Impression: The scene is safe for entry and exit. No injury is apparent on brief visual exam.

Initial Assessment:

Mental Status—A&O × 3, GCS 15.

Airway—Clear and patent at this time.

Breathing—Respirations 16.

Circulation—Radial pulse at 84 bpm.

Disability/Perfusion—Moves all four extremities, but reluctantly. Skin warm, dry, and pale.

Status after Initial Assessment: Serious, but stable.

Possible Differential (Field) Diagnoses: Gastroenteritis, appendicitis, ectopic pregnancy or ovarian, incarcerated hernia, regional ileitis, kidney stone, bowel obstruction, pelvic inflammatory disease, gastritis or PUD, pancreatitis, hepatitis, cholecystitis.

Initial Management Priorities: Oxygen at nasal cannula, cardiac monitor, IV access.

Focused History (SAMPLE):

Signs and Symptoms—Pale, warm, dry skin; lying on her side in distress; complains of being bloated and having diarrhea.

Allergies—Codeine.

Medications—None.

Past Medical History—Crohn's disease, but has not had problems in several years, tubal ligation two years ago. Last menstrual period 3–4 weeks ago, but is not sure. She is sexually active.

Last Oral Intake—The patient states that she had a large dinner with her family a few hours ago. If asked, no one else is ill at this time.

Events Preceding—The patient tells you that for the past few days, she has felt worn out, had a loss of appetite. She had ten bouts of diarrhea with abdominal cramping since eating a 3–4 hours ago.

OPQRST:

Onset—The pain came on very suddenly.

Palliation/Provocation—The cramping just seems to come and go.

Quality—Cramping pain in her lower abdomen. Worse on the left side.

Radiation—None.

Severity—On a scale of 1 to 10, it's a 6.

Time/Duration—Three to four hours.

Vital Signs:

Respirations—16 rapid and deep.

Pulse—Radial pulse 84 bpm.

Blood Pressure—116/76, slight increase in heart rate with orthostatic evaluation.

Temperature—98.4°F (37°C).

Pulse Oximetry—99%.

Blood Glucose Level—128 mg/dl.

Focused Physical Exam (Focused Medical Assessment): Lower-left quadrant abdominal pain diarrhea. Abdomen distended and tender to palpation. Stools liquid brown. No signs of bleeding. Normal urine. No vaginal discharge.

Differential/Field Diagnosis: Gastroenteritis, appendicitis, ectopic pregnancy or ovarian, incarcerated hernia, regional ileitis, kidney stone, bowel obstruction, diverticulitis pelvic inflammatory disease, food poisoning, or ulcerative colitis.

Management:

1) High-flow oxygen via nasal cannula.

2) IV access of NS or LR—fluid bolus acceptable. Titrate rate to BP.

3) Cardiac monitor.

4) Rapid transport to appropriate facility in position of comfort.

5) Analgesia not allowed by mouth.

Critical Actions:

1) Apply supplemental oxygen.

2) Place patient in a position of comfort.

3) IV access and monitor vital signs.

Teaching Points

1) There are numerous causes and etiologies of abdominal pain. Assist the participants in classifying the pain to body system and causes for rule outs.

2) Always follow an organized approach to rule out possible causes.

3) Any female of child-bearing age with abdominal pain should be considered to have an ectopic pregnancy until it is ruled out.

4) Be prepared to support vascular status.

5) Transport in position of comfort.

6) Discuss the possible differential/field diagnoses.

   ▶ Gastroenteritis—Possible, but keep other more life-threatening diagnoses on the list. The possibility of other GI problems is a much greater concern.

   ▶ Appendicitis—Possible, but not as likely due to pain location and severe diarrhea.

   ▶ Ectopic pregnancy or ovarian cyst (If female)—Possible, the severe diarrhea makes it questionable. Even though she has had a tubal ligation, it is still a possibility. Ectopic pregnancy pain is usually colicky. Monitor for radiation of pain to the shoulder. It would be important to keep this potential diagnosis on the list, due to the potential for rupture and bleeding, so frequent re-evaluation of hemodynamic status is indicated.

   ▶ Incarcerated hernia—Possible due to abdominal pain, but not likely due to severe diarrhea. Pain is usually more severe. Pain usually begins as crampy, then progresses to severe poorly localized pain. No mass noted. More common in males than females.

- Regional ileitis (Crohn's disease)—Most likely based on her history of Crohn's disease and diarrhea. The pain usually presents in the lower-right quadrant, but can present in other quadrants. Diverticulitis less likely due to age, but otherwise very similar.
- Kidney stone or infection—Possible, but not likely due to pain description and patient presentation.
- Bowel obstruction—Possible. The pain is consistent with a bowel obstruction and the patient has abdominal distention.
- Pelvic inflammatory disease—Possible due to history, but not as likely due to pain presentation and diarrhea
- Food poisoning—Possible due to presentation, but not as likely because no one else is ill.

Evaluation

1) *Excellent:* The participant's evaluation of the patient followed set format: initial assessment, focused history (SAMPLE, OPQRST) in an efficient manner. The participant displayed a thorough knowledge of the patient's condition, performed the exam and management in an organized manner, identified appropriate differential field diagnoses and demonstrated an excellent overall performance.

2) *Good:* The participant's evaluation of the patient followed set format: initial assessment, focused history (SAMPLE, OPQRST) in an acceptable manner with only minor deviation. The participant displayed an above-average knowledge of the patient's condition, performed the exam and management of the patient's condition, and demonstrated an above-average performance.

3) *Fair:* The participant's evaluation of the patient deviated from the set format without causing any further injury to the patient. The participant displayed an average or basic knowledge of the patient's condition and performed an adequate exam and management of the patient's condition.

4) *Inadequate:* The participant's evaluation of the patient deviated significantly from the set format, or the participant's actions endangered the patient's life or significantly exacerbated the condition.

▶ Acute Abdominal Pain/GI Bleeding: Scenario 4

Requirements: One instructor and one patient for every five participants.

Prerequisites: Read Chapter 8 "Acute Abdominal Pain"; Chapter 9 "Gastrointestinal Bleeding"; and Chapter 12 "Headache, Nausea, and Vomiting."

Equipment: One table and chair for the patient to use; jump kit with oxygen supplies (NC, NRM, aerosol mask, PPV device, intubation equipment), stethoscope, BP cuff, cardiac monitor, pulse oximeter (optional, but recommended), and medication kit with associated medications.

Instructor: Your role is vital because you must act as the coordinator of the station and also interact in the scenario. Before the participants arrive at the station, please review the scenario with your patient. Please read the scenario to become familiar with the necessary responses. Do not "coach" the participants along during the testing station; rather, allow them to conduct the exam without interruption or help.

Patient: One female (or male) patient. As the patient, you will be required to play the role of a 56-year-old female (or male) suffering from acute abdominal pain. You will be responsive and answer all questions. Please read the scenario to become familiar with the information.

Instructions

Hi, my name is _____, and I will be the examiner for this station. This is a hands-on patient assessment station. You will be given information concerning a patient experiencing a medical crisis. You will have all the necessary equipment you need to manage the patient in this station. Please look over the equipment before we go any further. You will be provided with pertinent information only when you ask the appropriate question. For any hands-on procedure, such as auscultation of a blood pressure or breath sounds or taking a pulse, select the appropriate equipment needed (if any) and use the equipment in the manner that it would be used on a patient. I will then give you the relevant clinical data. For example, you must select, place, and begin inflation of the BP cuff before the blood pressure is given to you. I will not answer questions in place of the patient. Therefore, it is imperative that you interact with your patient. Please verbalize to me any signs or symptoms that you find so that I will know you are cognizant of the patient and the patient's clinical appearance. The goal of this station is for you to complete an assessment with emphasis on the use of the SAMPLE and OPQRST history to develop a differential field diagnoses and initiate appropriate treatment.

Scenario

Advise the participants that they are responding to an abdominal pain call. If the participants are nurses or in-hospital providers, the scenario can be modified to the medical environment—such as the triage nurse brings a patient who complains of "upper abdominal pain" to Medical Room 1. The participant should use the assessment taught in this course.

Initial Impression: 56-year-old female lying on the bed. The patient is in obvious distress and cannot seem to find a position of comfort.

Scene Size-up/General Impression: The scene is safe for entry and exit. No injury is apparent on brief visual exam.

Initial Assessment:

    Mental Status—Responsive and alert to all commands

    Airway—Clear and patent at this time

    Breathing—Respirations 18 and shallow

    Circulation—Radial pulse strong at 88 bpm

    Disability/Perfusion—Moves all extremities frequently repositioning herself; pale, warm, dry skin

Status after Initial Assessment: Stable, potentially serious

Possible Differential (Field) Diagnoses: Gastric ulcers/gastritis, AMI, gallstones/cholecycstitis, kidney stones, pneumonia, pancreatitis

Initial Management Priorities: Oxygen therapy as tolerated by patient, cardiac monitor, IV access

Focused History (SAMPLE):

    Signs and Symptoms—Restless, upper-right quadrant abdominal pain.

    Allergies—Penicillin.

    Medications—Antacid, takes when her stomach is upset. Sometimes it helps.

    Past Medical History—Intermittent abdominal pain for past year but it always went away so the patient never had it "checked out."

    Last Oral Intake—Dinner a few hours ago.

    Events Preceding—The patient went out to dinner last night. After the patient arrived home last night, she developed abdominal pain. She spent most of the night pacing back and forth around the house, which alleviated the pain. The pain finally got better so she ate this morning and the pain is back.

OPQRST:

    Onset—It started last night after dinner.

    Palliation/Provocation—Walking around seems to make the pain better, but she is too tired to move.

    Quality—Cramping. It comes and goes.

    Radiation—The pain started here (pointing to upper-right quadrant) and goes into my back.

    Severity—On a scale of 1 to 10, it's an 8.

    Time/Duration—The patient went out to dinner last night. After the patient arrived home last night, she developed abdominal pain. She spent most of the night pacing back and forth around the house, which alleviated the pain. The pain finally got better so she ate this morning and the pain is back.

Vital Signs:

    Respirations—18 and shallow.

    Pulse—Radial pulse strong at 88 bpm.

    Blood Pressure—118/76.

    Temperature—98.2°F (36.8°C).

    Pulse Oximetry—99%.

    Blood Glucose Level—118 mg/dl

Focused Physical Exam (Focused Medical Assessment): Upper-right quadrant tenderness. Strong pulses in all extremities. Vomits breakfast (brown color); she tells you she had coffee and toast. No blood. Normal urine. Bowel movements are fluffy and lighter in color than usual.

Differential/Field Diagnosis: Gastric ulcers/gastritis, AMI, gallstones/cholecycstitis, kidney stones, pneumonia, aortic abdominal aneurysm, pancreatitis, hepatitis.

Management:

1) High-flow oxygen if tolerated.

2) IV access—rehydrate if needed

3) Monitor—12 lead ECG NSR. No abnormalities noted.

4) Transport to appropriate facility in position of comfort.

Critical Actions:

1) Assessing for possible life threats

Teaching Points

1) There are numerous causes and etiologies of abdominal pain. Assist the participants in classifying abdominal pain to body system and causes for rule outs.

2) Always follow an organized approach to rule out possible causes.

3) Don't let scene clues lead you to a diagnosis preemptively.

4) Discuss visceral versus parietal pain.

5) Discuss the possible differential/field diagnoses

   ▶ Gastric ulcers/gastritis—Possible, due to history gastric pain with antacid relief, but not as likely the problem because gastritis tends to present as a burning pain and not a continuous cramping pain.

   ▶ AMI—Possible, but history indicates another cause. It would be important to keep this potential diagnosis on the list, due to the stress the patient is experiencing. Even though the ECG is negative, damage may still be a potential, so cardiac monitoring should be considered.

   ▶ Gallstones/cholecystitis—Very likely due to pain presentation. Pain occurred after eating. Pain was colicky and radiated to the back, which is consistent with gall stones. In addition, movement and pacing seemed to relieve the pain.

   ▶ Kidney stone or infection—Possible, but not as likely as gallstones. The pain is colicky, but not in the flank area. The patient has no urinary problems.

   ▶ Left lung pneumonia—Not likely due to clear lungs sounds and no recent respiratory involvement.

   ▶ Aortic abdominal aneurysm—Possible due to pain radiating to the back, but not likely due to crampy description of the pain and no other indications.

Evaluation

1) *Excellent:* The participant's evaluation of the patient followed set format: initial assessment, focused history (SAMPLE, OPQRST) in an efficient manner. The participant displayed a thorough knowledge of the patient's condition, performed the exam and management in an organized manner, identified appropriate differential field diagnoses, and demonstrated an excellent overall performance.

2) *Good:* The participant's evaluation of the patient followed set format: initial assessment, focused history (SAMPLE, OPQRST) in an acceptable manner with only minor deviation. The participant displayed an above-average knowledge of the patient's condition, performed the exam and management of the patient's condition, and demonstrated an above-average performance.

3) *Fair:* The participant's evaluation of the patient deviated from the set format without causing any further injury to the patient. The participant displayed an average or basic knowledge of the patient's condition and performed an adequate exam and management of the patient's condition.

4) *Inadequate:* The participant's evaluation of the patient deviated significantly from the set format, or the participant's actions endangered the patient's life or significantly exacerbated the condition.

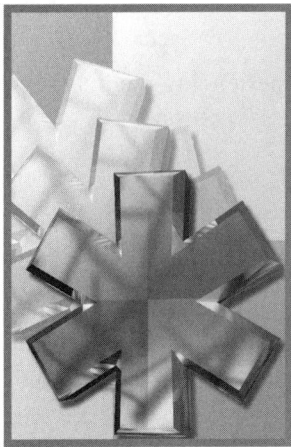

V. ADVANCED MEDICAL LIFE SUPPORT PROVIDER COURSE SLIDE NOTES

CHAPTER 1: ASSESSMENT OF THE MEDICAL PATIENT

SLIDE NO.   **SLIDE TITLE/NOTES**

Slide 1-1   **The National Association of EMTs (NAEMT)**
The AMLS Provider course is sponsored by the NAEMT. The course is endorsed by NAEMSP.

Slide 1-2   **AMLS Provider Course Objectives**
Discuss course objectives.

Slide 1-3   **AMLS Provider Course Objectives**
Discuss course objectives.

Slide 1-4   **Successful Course Completion**
- ▶ Attendance at both days is required. The AMLS course completion certificate and wallet card will be awarded. Active participation by the participants is required for all lecture and practical station scenarios. This course is an interactive, scenario-based presentation of various medical emergencies. The course is designed to enhance the knowledge and skills of the healthcare professionals who encounter patients with a variety of medical emergencies.
- ▶ A team leader approach is used throughout the course. Live patients will be used for practical scenarios. Successful completion ensures participants are awarded 16 hours of CME. This course can be used for the medical CME for the National Registry of EMTs (NREMT) recognition.

Slide 1-5   **AMLS Course History**
Currently, 12,500 providers, 1,500 instructors, and 120 affiliate faculty are trained (4/1/06).

Slide 1-6   **Assessment of the Medical Patient—Chapter 1**
- ▶ Many major medical emergencies may not be definitively managed in the prehospital environment. A comprehensive assessment and early recognition of lifethreats for patients experiencing medical emergencies will improve outcomes by all healthcare providers. Competency in a rapid, accurate assessment ensures effective, efficient patient care and

more positive outcomes. Patients experiencing medical emergencies can often have subtle presentations of signs/symptoms.

Slide 1-7   **The AMLS Assessment**
- ▶ Early recognition and management of potential or actual lifethreats is essential for all healthcare providers. At the scene, focused history and diagnostic information is obtained and management of the patient is altered. Assessment and management of the patient continues to be assessed and altered until care is transferred to the receiving facility. For the purposes of this course, differential (field) diagnoses are identified by all levels of healthcare practitioners. These diagnoses determine management strategies. Active listening and communication skills, along with good critical thinking skills, are essential in obtaining comprehensive patient information from patients experiencing medical emergencies.

Slide 1-8   **The Initial Assessment**
- ▶ The initial assessment information reveals the possible underlying etiologies/diagnoses.

Slide 1-9   **The AMLS Assessment**
- ▶ The physical exam, vital signs, and focused history components of the assessment narrow the possibilities to probabilities. Continued evaluation of lifethreats and changes in management strategies are ongoing throughout the duration of care for the patient. In a responsive medical patient, the focused medical assessment concentrates on the body systems/area of chief complaint. In an unresponsive patient, a rapid medical assessment is performed. This is a quick head-to-toe assessment, similar to a rapid trauma assessment. Inspection, palpation, auscultation, and percussion for evidence of abnormal findings are done to identify the severity of the instability and rule-in and rule-out potential and probable differential (field) diagnoses.
- ▶ The assessment-based approach of the initial assessment identifies and corrects life-threatening emergencies.

Slide 1-10   **Global Assessment**
- ▶ Scene stability is crucial to the safety of patients and healthcare providers. BSI considerations are infectious disease from tears, amniotic fluid, oozing lesions, urine, saliva, vomit, feces, and viruses such as TB and MRSA (methicillin-resistant staphylococcus aureus). Don't rule out that a medical patient may have also experienced a trauma and viceversa. Bystanders and family members can provide critical information on preceding events or medical history for an unconscious patient.
- ▶ Identifying environmental concerns can determine rapid movement of the patient out of the environment and initiation of emergent treatment. Improperly clothed for the temperature; exertion in hot, humid weather; not heating or cooling their environment appropriately are environmental concerns.

▶ Information gathered here can determine packaging of the patient and access in or out of the environment.

▶ This is the first component of the assessment-based approach to patient care.

Slide 1-11   **What Is the Scene Telling You?**

▶ Noises—Audible adventitious breath sounds and domestic disputes can be ominous.

▶ Odors—Incontinence, musty breath (liver disease), fruity-breath (DKA), toxic fumes, alcohol intoxication, decubitus ulcers, and infection are all indications of altered mentation and poor perfusion.

▶ Medicine containers/prescribed/OTC—Multiple medication containers can indicate drug toxicity or noncompliance. Evaluation of this evidence can indicate drug dependency and multiple disease processes.

▶ Assistive devices—Can give clues on chronic versus acute disease pathologies. Oxygen concentrators/nebulizer equipment is used for COPD, cystic fibrosis, asthma, and cancer patients. Walkers, canes, wheelchairs, and prosthetics indicate chronic poor perfusion.

▶ Hunches—Use your experience, attitude, and knowledge of anatomy and physiology and disease processes to heighten awareness of the environment, and patient global presentation to determine lifethreats and early management strategies.

▶ Exposure to biological, chemical, and nuclear agents used by terrorists must be assessed when responding to medical emergencies. Nerve agents, like Sarin and Tabun, bind with cholinesterase, leading to excess acetycholine, inhibiting nerve transmission. Patients present with salivation, lacrimation, urination, defecation, and emesis (SLUDGE) pinpoint pupils, bronchoconstriction, laryngospasm, altered mental status, and seizures. Visual disturbances, muscle cramps, and diaphoresis are common. Aerosol exposures take seconds to minutes; liquid agents minutes to hours to present.

Slide 1-12   **Global Assessment**

▶ Patient age, gender, or ethnicity can indicate potential ectopic pregnancy, hemophilia, sickle-cell anemia, and differences in presentation of AMI. Facial and body affect assists in identifying mental status and CNS difficulty.

▶ Assesses whether the patient is awake and/or alert. Can indicate sick or not sick, fear, anxiousness, and pain. Body positioning can indicate severity of patient presentation. This assessment identifies patient packaging and transport concerns.

Slide 1-13   **Global Assessment**

▶ Flexion—Stroke, subdural hematoma, encephalitis, or meningitis. Assess for history of recent fall, especially in the elderly.

▶ Extension—Brain stem injury that indicates a more severe CNS injury.

	SLIDE NO.	SLIDE TITLE/NOTES

Slide 1-14 **Initial Assessment**
- ▶ All the components of the initial assessment are part of the AMLS assessment-based approach.

Slide 1-15 **Airway Assessment**
- ▶ Physical obstructions should be removed according to current American Heart Association guidelines. Snoring may indicate the tongue is an obstruction. Gurgling indicates fluid in the upper airway, stridor indicates partial upper airway obstruction, rales indicate fluid, crowing and hoarseness indicate obstruction due to a foreign body or edema. Evaluate airway for vomitus, secretions, blood, edema, or signs of anaphylaxis. A compromised airway requires immediate intervention.

Slide 1-16 **Airway Management**
- ▶ Manual maneuvers—Head tilt, head tilt-chin lift, modified jaw thrust, or tongue-jaw lift.
- ▶ Suction—soft or rigid devices should be used as deemed appropriate.
- ▶ Healthcare providers should use basic interventions before advanced interventions for airway management. Dual lumen devices may include: LMA® or Combitube®. Tracheal intubation should be considered as a definitive airway in all patients that are unable to maintain their own airway. Transtracheal jet ventilation could be considered in patients that have laryngeal edema, such as what is related to anaphylaxis. Surgical cricothyrotomy and transtracheal jet ventilation are techniques that require high levels of skill and competence.

Slide 1-17 **Breathing Assessment**
- ▶ Increased respiratory rates decrease tidal volume and promote hypoxia. Poor tidal volume decreases alveolar ventilation and leads to poor gas exchange sooner than a slower rate. Retractions of the intercostal spaces, suprasternal notch, supraclavicular spaces, and subcostal area and asymmetric chest wall movement are indications of instability. Stridor indicates partial upper airway obstruction from edema or foreign body; snoring indicates the tongue may be blocking the airway. Gurgling and rales indicate fluid in the upper airway.

Slide 1-18 **Breathing Assessment**
- ▶ Irregular breathing patterns such as Kussmaul's are related to DKA and acidosis. This type of respiratory pattern is an attempt to compensate for elimination of CO_2 seen in DKA and toxic ingestion. The Cheyne-Stokes crescendo-decrescendo with periods of apnea is related to CNS dysfunction and brain injury. Biot's and central neurogenic hyperventilation are related to brain injury secondary to stroke, hepatic failure, electrolyte imbalance, and intracranial infection.

Slide 1-19 **Breathing Assessment**
- ▶ Decreases in tidal volume decrease alveolar ventilation.

Slide 1-20 **Breathing Management**

▶ The healthcare provider must consider which supplemental oxygen device will deliver the appropriate oxygen concentration to meet the patient's needs. Positive pressure ventilation should be done at a normal ventilation rate for an adult patient. Hyperventilation is discouraged for patients with increased intracerebral pressure. Needle decompression is used for presentations of tension pneumothorax. Oxygen saturation should be continually monitored before and after supplemental oxygen.

Slide 1-21 **Circulation Assessment**

▶ Assess the regularity and quality of central and peripheral pulses. Weak peripheral pulses indicate hypotension and possible cardiac dysfunction. Pulse strength is a clue to volume and hydration status. Irregular pulses are a clue to dysrhythmias. Dysrhythmias can be caused by hypoxia, toxic ingestion, and electrolyte disturbances. Pulse rates that are too fast or too slow should be identified. Tachycardia/bradycardia may result in decreased cardiac output and decreased perfusion. Major bleeds result from esophaegeal varices, vaginal and gastrointestinal disorders, varicose veins, past surgeries, and epistaxis. Perfusion assessments may also be done during the evaluation of the circulation status.

Slide 1-22 **Circulation Assessment**

Slide 1-23 **Circulation Management**

▶ Manage internal and external blood loss with the administration of isotonic IV solutions, such as normal saline. Positioning a patient supine or trendelenberg will assist with inhibiting poor perfusion from blood loss. Rapid and careful packaging and transport of patients exhibiting blood loss is critical to maintaining stability. In cases of cardiogenic shock, dopamine or dobutamine may be interventions that are considered.

Slide 1-24 **Disability/Perfusion Assessment**

▶ The AVPU scale should be used to determine the level of consciousness. This scale evaluates cognition and orientation. Unresponsiveness is always an indication of instability and an immediate life threat. Observe for posturing associated with increasing intracranial pressure. Use alert to person, place, and time to determine awareness and awakeness. Awareness indicates cerebral hemispheres are intact and the reticular activating system (RAS) is functioning. RAS obtains sensory information and sends it to the thalamus, the editor of the brain, for interpretation. Neuronal messages are sent to the cerebral hemispheres to react to messages from the RAS (physical, emotional, verbal). Moaning and groaning may indicate diminished consciousness and pain. Cognitive impairment is a potential indicator of intracranial pressure, seizure, CVA, electrolyte imbalance, hypoxia, hypovolemia, thiamine deficiency, hypothermia, and infection. Capillary refill can be unreliable in adult patients, but

	SLIDE NO.	SLIDE TITLE/NOTES

should be evaluated. Skin should be evaluated for color, temperature, and moisture. A Glasgow Coma Scale (GCS) should be done on every medical patient.

Slide 1-25   **Perfusion Assessment**

► Elderly with vascular disease can have unreliable capillary refills. A perfusion assessment is critical in determining if your patient is physiologically stable versus unstable.

Slide 1-26   **Perfusion Assessment**

► Hot skin indicates fever, infection, and heat emergencies. Cold skin indicates shock, cold emergencies, and hypothermia. Cyanosis is a late sign of hypoxia. Red or flushed skin indicates vasodilation of peripheral vessels related to overdose (OD), anaphylaxis, poisoning, neurogenic shock with spine injury, inflammation, DKA, fever, or extreme thermal emergencies. Mottled, blotchy skin indicates cardiovascular compromise and poor perfusion. Extremely dry skin indicates severe dehydration, drug OD, or poisoning.

Slide 1-27   **Disability/Perfusion Assessment**

► Key components to the GCS are eye opening, motor response, and verbal response. GCS provides a uniform system for determining a patient's level of consciousness. This scale has more prognostic value and is more discriminating that AVPU. Two indicators of physiological instability are no spontaneous eye opening and no movement to painful stimuli. Evaluate speech patterns for usage of few words before gasping breaths, which indicates severity. A GCS less than 8 indicates coma and the need to aggressively protect the airway, a GCS of 7–8 has a 94% positive outcome, and a GCS of 3–4 has a 10% positive outcome.

Slide 1-28   **Global/Initial Assessment Priorities**

► Aggressive airway management, drug administration, IV therapy, and continuous cardiac monitoring should be initiated. This determination is made at any time during the A, B, C, perfusion assessment and/or at the conclusion of the initial assessment.

Slide 1-29   **Establishing Physiological Instability**

► Prehospital personnel will use these priorities to initiate rapid interventions and transport. In-house personnel have internal protocols to establish teams which may consist of a house supervisor and ICU/CCU RN or intern who evaluates patients that begin to decompensate so that emergent care can begin prior to contacting the physician or needing to begin resuscitation. Evaluation of all the possibilities of differential (field) diagnoses should be done upon completion of the initial assessment.

Slide 1-30   **Focused History and Medical Assessment**

► In a responsive patient, the history is done first, followed by the physical exam and vital signs. In an unresponsive patient, the physical exam and vital signs are performed before the history. When gathering a history, questions should be presented in either open-ended or closed-ended formats to the patient, depending on their degree of discomfort or mentation.

Slide 1-31 **Baseline Vital Signs**
▸ In an unstable patient, take a blood pressure in both extremities. SpO_2 readings less than 95% warrant oxygen therapy, unless contraindicated. The rate, quality, and rhythm of the respirations should be assessed. An evaluation of lung sounds is essential. Determining the quality, regularity, and rate of the pulse is done here. Cardiac arrhythmias should be treated per AHA guidelines. Patients with altered mentation should have pupils continually checked to rule out toxicity, seizure, and stroke. Determining a baseline blood glucose level is essential.

Slide 1-32 **SAMPLE—Past Medical History**
▸ If responsive, the patient is the best historian to obtain a focused history. If unresponsive, bystanders and family are resources that can be used for this information.
  S S/s the patient is presenting with the possibilities of diagnoses you have determined at this point in your assessment. Previous surgeries and exposure to chemicals, smoke, toxins, or infectious disease should be determined.
  A Allergies to medications (newly prescribed/OTC) or foods.
  M Medications (prescription and OTC).
  P Past medical history may include hypertension, respiratory conditions, diabetes, or stroke. Determine when they have last seen a physician.
  L Liquid or solid food intake is important if surgery is pending and alerts the practitioner to risk of vomiting.
  E Determining if the patient was at rest or exerting themselves can indicate severity and whether a gradual or sudden onset.

Slide 1-33 **Focused History**
▸ Familial and social history information may indicate occupational hazards and concerns to inform the receiving facility personnel or physician.
▸ Determining the activity level of the patient is important when evaluating chronic diseases and transport modalities.

Slide 1-34 **Focused History**
▸ Determining associated complaints is essential in ruling in and ruling out body systems and differential (field) diagnoses.

Slide 1-35 **OPQRST–Present Illness History**
▸ Present illness related to the chief complaint is obtained.
  O When did the s/s start? Was there a sudden or gradual onset?
  P What makes the discomfort/pain better or worse? What relief measures has the patient done? Example: taking OTC medications.
  Q Have patient describe the quality of the discomfort/pain. Descriptions like crampy, dull, sharp, achy, crushing, knifelike, and pressure can assist the practitioner in

determining the body organ or system that is causing the discomfort/pain. This early identification can prompt more rapid interventions.

R Does the discomfort/pain stay in one location or does it move? Referred pain, such as knee pain for a hip injury, can indicate the severity and perfusion compromise.

S Using a scale of 0–10, a patient should rate the discomfort/pain. If a patient is unable to verbalize this information, the Wong-Baker FACES Pain Rating Scale can be used.

T Is the duration of the discomfort/pain an issue for the patient? Determining what makes it more significant at this time can help the provider determine severity or possibly an exacerbation of a chronic condition.

Slide 1-36   **Focused History—Discomfort/Pain Radiation**

Slide 1-37   **Focused Medical Assessment**

▶ In patients with good level of consciousness, the area of chief complaint is evaluated. A look, listen, and feel approach is used. If the patient is unresponsive, a head-to-toe exam is done. Life threats are identified and managed as they are found. Treatment modalities are monitored or altered to accommodate patient need and new findings. In patients with diminished mentation, a thorough neurological exam would be done. This exam includes: pupils, distal pulses, capillary refill, and motor and sensory evaluations.

Slide 1-38   **Focused Medical Assessment**

▶ Assess nerves II, III, IV, and VI by looking at pupil reaction to light and extraoccular movement of looking up, down, and to the right and left. Normal speech tests nerves IX, X, and XII. Nerve VII can be evaluated by having the patient smile and raise both eyebrows. Clenching teeth assesses nerve V. Nerve VIII is checked by having the patient cover one ear with their hand and attempt to detect a whisper. Nerve XI is assessed by having the patient shrug his or her shoulders. Cincinnati Stroke Scale can be used: 1) smile showing teeth, 2) close eyes and hold both arms out in front for 10 seconds to evaluate pronator drift, and 3) speech evaluation by asking the patient to say, "You can't teach an old dog new tricks." The Los Angeles scale uses the above and evaluates age, history of seizure/epilepsy, duration of symptoms, mobility, and blood glucose levels. Detailed physical exams and ongoing assessments are continuous evaluation of the patient's response to treatment modalities and can depend on transport times for prehospital personnel.

Slide 1-39   **Management Strategies**

Slide 1-40   **Possibilities to Probabilities**

▶ Obtaining vital signs, focused history, and focused medical assessments moves the assessment-based approach to a diagnostic-based approach to identify and treat underlying diagnoses.

Slide 1-41   **Scenario 1**

▶ This patient is unstable and should require more urgent evaluation and prompt patient room assignment. What do we know about her presentation? She is sick with potential airway compromise and altered mentation.

Slide 1-42   **Initial Assessment—Scenario 1**

▶ Patient is unstable and a potential life threat. Immediate interventions are to move her to an exam room in a lateral recumbant position with supplemental oxygen via nasal cannula.

Slide 1-43   **Initial Assessment—Scenario 1**

▶ Instability is confirmed.

Slide 1-44   **Initial Assessment—Scenario 1**

▶ Patient is unstable. Oxygen, blood glucose levels, oxygen saturation, cardiac monitor, IV therapy, and temperature are emergent treatments. Possible differential diagnoses: altered mental status related to endocrine abnormality, electrolyte imbalance, infection, hypovolemia, OD/poisoning, DKA/hyperglycemia, intracranial infection, or internal bleeding from ectopic pregnancy.

Slide 1-45   **Baseline Vital Signs—Scenario 1**

▶ What is the significance of high blood sugar in this scenario? The elevated blood sugar in ASA overdose is not always present, but represents the net balance between induced glycolysis and inhibition of gluconeogenesis and increased consumption. Brain glucose is often low despite mild elevation in serum glucose so the objective is to keep the blood glucose level on the high side. If very high, will contribute to dehydration. Hyperventilation increases CO_2 excretion leading to respiratory alkalosis. This excites neurons and can cause agitation and muscle twitching. This activity uses cellular ATP and increases lactic acid which can precipitate metabolic acidosis.

Slide 1-46   **Focused History—SAMPLE Scenario 1**

Slide 1-47   **Focused History—OPQRST Scenario 1**

▶ What differential diagnoses can be determined? Aggressive doses of antipyretics and the headache are important information.

Slide 1-48   **Focused Medical Assessment—Scenario 1**

▶ Flexion of the neck that causes pain and involuntary flexion of the hips while the patient is supine is known as Brudzinski's sign. This sign may be absent in the elderly. If the hips flex during a nuchal flexion maneuver, it is an indication of diffuse meningeal irritation in the spinal nerve root. A nuchal maneuver is done when a hand is placed under the head of the patient and the provider tries to flex the neck by moving it forward.

▶ Kernig's sign is another indicator of meningeal irritation. To perform this exam, a practitioner will place the patient supine and flex the hip and knees on one side and then extend the knee while the hip is still flexed. The patient will resist extension of the knee. Both signs can be indications of encephalitis and meningitis.

▶ Why the nystagmus, twitching, high blood sugar, low potassium, and metabolic acidosis with quiet tachypnea? The acid-base status depends on the net balance of primary respiratory alkalosis (which usually predominates early), mixed metabolic alkalosis (due to dehydration), and metabolic acidosis (due to anaerobic and generally increased metabolism which generally predominates late).

Slide 1-49   **Differential Diagnoses—Scenario 1**

Slide 1-50   **Additional History Information—Scenario 1**
▶ This is an extremely high dose of aspirin for her weight. Mild to moderate toxicity with 150 mg/kg and severe with 150–300 mg/kg.

Slide 1-51   **Differential DX—Salicylate Toxicity—Scenario 1**
▶ Salicylate toxicity affects the CNS. The fever is the result of the acute pharyngitis that led to the excess ASA intake.

Slide 1-52   **Salicylate Overdose Management—Scenario 1**
▶ Supplemental potassium administration if levels are low and expect to go lower to correct acidemia.

Slide 1-53   **Summary**

Slide 1-54   **Summary**

Slide 1-55   **Summary**

CHAPTER 2: AIRWAY MANAGEMENT, VENTILATION, AND OXYGEN THERAPY

SLIDE   **SLIDE TITLE/NOTES**

Slide 2-1   **Airway Management and Ventilation**
- ▶ Airway is a common topic in healthcare education but still the most commonly mismanaged part of emergency care.
- ▶ Oxygen is the key to human life and its main route into the body is the airway.
- ▶ We will presume that your previous education has familiarized you to basic airway management. We will review:
  - — Respiratory anatomy and physiology
  - — Basic and advanced airway adjuncts
  - — Medication-assisted intubation
  - — Failed intubation plans
  - — Ventilation techniques

Slide 2-2   **Assessment of the Airway**
- ▶ The healthcare provider must ask some simple questions while evaluating the airway.
- ▶ Medical assessment begins with scene evaluation, an across-the-room assessment of the patient, and then evaluation of the ABCs.
- ▶ Airway assessment begins with a simple conversation in which the healthcare provider introduces him/herself and asks how the patient is. If the patient converses without difficulty, the airway should be patent.
- ▶ If the patient converses with difficulty or does not speak, a more intensive assessment of airway must be initiated. Look for reasons that may threaten the patient's airway: tongue, teeth, blood, secretions, vomitus, etc. Immediate resuscitation of airway threats must take place prior to assessment of the patient's respiratory status.

Slide 2-3   **Airway Interventions**
- ▶ Additional logistical questions asked while treating any compromised airway.
- ▶ If airway maneuvers need to be performed, the healthcare provider must use basic airway interventions initially and, if an advanced healthcare provider, the organization of future airway needs are based on scope of practice and the situation (e.g., how far away from the hospital are we?).
- ▶ How difficult might it be to intubate this patient?

Slide 2-4   **Indications for Airway Management**
- ▶ Alteration in mental status:
  - — Watch carefully for and provide management of the airway.
  - — The most common mistake made in airway management is failure to recognize when a patient who is breathing on his/her own BUT has altered mental status and needs airway adjuncts to PROTECT the airway.
- ▶ Hypoxia:
  - — The patient in respiratory distress who may be in respiratory failure progresses easily into arrest.

— Aggressive ventilatory management with airway adjuncts may be needed.
▶ Medical emergency:
— Anticipate that in some medical conditions the patient may need airway management. Be prepared.
— Angioedema and infections are some examples.

Slide 2-5   **Review of Basic Airway Techniques**
▶ Review the basic airway maneuvers as shown with indications, contraindications, and techniques.

Slide 2-6   **Advanced/Alternative Airway Devices**
▶ These devices are generally termed "bridge" airways because they bridge the patient to intubation. There are many new devices on the market and the healthcare provider should become familiar with several backup devices to intubation.
▶ These advanced airways do not require direct visualization. This is an introductory slide for the next three slides.
▶ These are categorized by their style or anatomic location: dual-lumen or supraglottic.

Slide 2-7   **Pharyngotracheal Lumen (PtL)® Airway**
▶ Dual-lumen (longer tube within a shorter tube) with a stylet and a large oropharyngeal cuff, blindly inserted. Describe the use of this device. Reinforce that attaching the strap around patient's head is essential in proper positioning of this device.
▶ Device is contraindicated in caustic ingestion and known esophageal disease.

Slide 2-8   **Esophageal Tracheal Combitube Airway®**
▶ Diagram showing the Combitube® in both the esophageal and tracheal positions.
▶ Similar to the PtL® but the dual-lumen tubes are side-by-side with a cuff on each tube.
▶ Describe the use of this device. The Combitube® has the same indications and contraindications as the PtL®. Emphasize that it requires the same skills and practice as the PtL®.

Slide 2-9   **King LT Airway or Device**
▶ This supraglottic device is an easy-to-insert and use single-lumen airway that has a color-coded system for sizes and dual cuffs that inflate simultaneously with one syringe (color coded to the top of the device). First introduced within research areas in 2005, is now fully approved by the FDA and being used by many EMS programs.

Slide 2-10   **Laryngeal Mask Airway (LMA)®**
▶ This is another supraglottic airway. Blindly inserted and used in multiple sizes for all age groups. As with any airway device, skill acquisition and retention is required.
▶ Like all supraglottic airways, this bridges to endotracheal intubation and does not protect the patient from aspiration of gastric contents.
▶ This slide includes some step-by-step activities for correct placement of the device.

SLIDE NO.	SLIDE TITLE/NOTES	NOTES

Slide 2-11 **Advanced Airway Procedures**
▶ Each technique will be discussed on the following slides.

Slide 2-12 **Quality Assurance for Endotracheal Intubation**
▶ Advanced healthcare providers who are credentialed to provide endotracheal intubation should assure themselves enough practice in this technique in order to become proficient, especially if considering using medications to enhance patient compliance.
▶ In order to maintain proficiency in this skill, performing 6–12 intubations per year (adult) is a minimum recommendation from the American Heart Association and the Society for Anesthesiology.

Slide 2-13 **LMA-Fastrach®**
▶ The LMA-Fastrach® is a specially designed LMA that allows an 8.0 mm ETT to be inserted without visualization. Insertion technique is similar to the LMA-Unique but the stainless steel adaptor guides blind ETT insertion.
▶ This device requires skill and practice—preferably in the operating room under the guidance of an anesthesiologist.

Slide 2-14 **Nasotracheal Intubation**
▶ Review the pros and cons.
▶ Use of this technique is appropriate as an alternative to orotracheal intubation when the patient:
— Cannot be placed into a supine position
— Is lethargic but not unconscious
— Has difficulties with swelling or secretions in the oropharynx (inhibits visualization)
— Has a clenched jaw
▶ This technique, however, does require skill and practice. Patient must be breathing. Success rate is fairly low and soft-tissue injury usually occurs.
▶ Delayed consequences of nasotracheal intubation:
— Small tubes (remember, the smaller the diameter of the tube, the more airway compromise)
— Complication rates higher

Slide 2-15 **Digital and Lighted-Stylet Intubation**
▶ Both techniques are essentially "blind" in that direct visualization is not performed.
▶ Lighted stylet:
— ET tube with lighted stylet advanced into larynx.
— Neck must be shielded from light source.
— Less risk to the healthcare provider than digital.
▶ Digital technique:
— Historically, the first way we intubated.
— Patient MUST be without any gag reflex.
— Epiglottis is palpated as 2 to 3 fingers are inserted into lower oropharynx (walk down the tongue).
— ETT (with stylet shaped into hockey stick or L) inserted behind fingers—2nd finger traps progressing ETT and guides it above identified epiglottis. Stop at intervals and remove portions of inserted stylet as you advance ETT distally.

	SLIDE NO.	SLIDE TITLE/NOTES

Slide 2-16 **Lighted-Stylet Intubation**
▶ A review of the steps. Note the placement of the fingers and the need to adapt this skill for digital intubation without stylet.

Slide 2-17 **Alternative Airways: Surgical**
▶ This is an introductory slide. These techniques are described in subsequent slides.
▶ Indications for surgical airway:
— ETT cannot be achieved
— Anatomic deformities (previous head/neck surgery)
— Direct obstruction of upper airway (edema foreign body airway obstruction [FBAO])

NOTE: Discussing these techniques does not authorize their use. Many regions do not allow EMS to provide these techniques.

Slide 2-18 **Surgical Airways: Percutaneous Transtracheal Jet Ventilation**
▶ High-pressure oxygen driven into the tracheobronchial tree as a TEMPORARY or bridge to a more definitive airway
— The problem is CO_2 retention.
— Limit of 30–45 minutes for this ventilation technique
— Need at least 50 psi to deliver the oxygen and ventilate
— Many modifications used to provide tubing with ventilation ports (including manufactured products)
— Complications include bleeding and hematoma formation, esophageal entrance with contamination of the mediastinum, infection, further airway compromise, damage to the thyroid gland, and subcutaneous emphysema

Slide 2-19 **Surgical Airways: Retrograde Intubation**
▶ The same anatomic location must be identified with this procedure as with percutaneous needle insufflation.
▶ In this technique, the needle is angled towards the head.
▶ A 24-inch+ J-wire is required and inserted through properly inserted needle until it can be visualized in the patient's mouth. Grasp wire with clamp and pull up and out of mouth, but DO NOT pull end of wire completely out of the needle.
▶ Insert guide wire through eye of distal ETT and pull ETT through mouth and into position where resistance is met near glottis.
▶ As guide wire is removed, apply gentle downward pressure on distal tip of positioned ETT to guide it into vocal cords. Inflate cuff of ETT and confirm placement.
▶ Retrograde intubation requires a great deal of dexterity, skill, and time.

Slide 2-20 **Surgical Cricothyrotomy**
▶ The recommended skin incision is made in the longitudinal plane to allow for more visual and physical access to the cricothyroid membrane and to decrease the risk of bleeding, where a small incision may then be made anatomically.

NOTE: This may be a procedure that is not allowed in your EMS region. The healthcare provider should consider BVM ventilation until the patient can be delivered to the resources necessary to provide this advanced airway technique in a more controlled environment.

▶ Steps to surgical cricothyrotomy:
— Insert ETT into surgical incision. ETT should be sized 1 mm less than would normally be inserted orotracheally.
— Must maintain patency of surgical incision with either a finger, clamp, etc. while ETT inserted. You may use commercially available devices, according to directions.
— Complications include hemorrhage, infection, etc.

Slide 2-21   Assessment of Ventilation

▶ Once the patient's airway is open, assess the patient's minute volume. Assess general rate and work of breathing:
— Quiet tachypnea (fast but not labored) is a sign of sympathetic nervous stimulation, such as shock.
— Labored breathing may be an indication of many major life-threatening illnesses.

▶ Once a sense of the patient's rate and work of breathing is assessed, assess the patient's tidal volume—is it adequate? Auscultation of breath sounds in the apices helps determine that air is moving in the lower airways and the patient is taking deep enough breaths for adequate tidal volume.

▶ For those patients presenting with extremes in respiratory rates (bradypnea, tachypnea) or with poor tidal volume, assisted ventilation may need to be provided.

▶ As you are assessing the patient in the initial assessment, the use of monitoring devices is not advisable. Once the focused exam is initiated, cardiac and respiratory monitoring devices can be used to help gather data about the patient's overall status. These devices, by themselves, are not to be used to determine whether a patient needs to have assisted ventilation or oxygen therapy.

Slide 2-22   Capnography

▶ In addition to cardiac monitoring and pulse oximetry, capnography may be a monitoring tool in the assessment of the patient's respiratory status.

▶ Colormetric devices vs. capnography with waveform technology must be evaluated by your healthcare service for the type that is appropriate for your environment. No matter which type of carbon dioxide detection technology is chosen, all types must be understood fully by healthcare providers.

Slide 2-23   Ventilation Equipment and Techniques

▶ Techniques listed on the slide:
— BVM (bag-value mask) with 2–3 people AND cricoid pressure (discussed in next two slides). Mimic a natural inspiratory and expiratory cycle when ventilating the patient via BVM.
— CPAP (continuous positive airway pressure) is positive pressure applied throughout the respiratory cycle to the spontaneously breathing patient with reliable ventilatory drive and adequate tidal volume. This device enhances oxygenation to the patient, similar to PEEP and ventilation.

> - Non-invasive pressure support ventilation (NIPSV) with separate pressure levels for inspiration and expiration is known as BiPAP (bilevel positive airway pressure).
> — Flow-restricted, oxygen-powered devices and techniques should again mimic a natural inspiratory/expiratory cycle and there is no indication of lung compliance with this device.
> — Pocket mask with supplemental oxygen and positive pressure may actually provide better tidal volume and less barotrauma than other devices.
> — One-person BVM is very difficult and may be the least effective method.

NOTE: Discuss these methods but reinforce the fact that all techniques should not cause high-pressure, forceful inspiratory phases with no chance at exhalation (which should be at least at a 1:2 ratio). All positive pressure ventilation without a protected airway will cause gastric insufflation unless precautions are taken.

Slide 2-24 | **Basic Ventilation Procedures**
> ▶ Pocket mask (as discussed on previous slide) usually provides better tidal volume than use of BVM, especially if used by only one rescuer. Adding supplemental oxygen to the pocket-mask device adds to this basic ventilation tool for a single rescuer.
> ▶ In BVM ventilation, ideally one rescuer provides a mask seal on the patient's face (emergency contraption [EC] clamp technique) and another rescuer provides positive pressure ventilation at a rate of 10–12 per minute for the adult. Adding supplemental oxygen and oxygen reservoir devices enhance oxygenation to the patient while providing ventilation.
> ▶ Cricoid pressure should be provided during all positive pressure ventilations in order to prevent passive regurgitation.

Slide 2-25 | **Ventilation**
> ▶ This slide reinforces the "slow and low" ventilation procedures advocated for BVM and updated to coincide with new AHA recommendations, 2005. It is important for all healthcare practitioners to avoid hyperventilation (too fast or too many). Each ventilation must be longer than 1 second, yet only enough to allow for visible chest rise at a reduced rate over past recommendations.
> ▶ This slide mentions hyperventilation techniques that may be used for the patient exhibiting signs of cerebral herniation in the late stages of increased intracranial pressure processes.
> ▶ Note that the rate of ventilation increases only to 15–20 per minute for this treatment. It should be guided by end-tidal CO_2 monitoring whenever available because a very narrow range of CO_2 is allowed for this practice.

Slide 2-26 | **Cricoid Pressure/Sellick's Maneuver**
> ▶ Landmarks of the anatomy.
> ▶ Use the thyroid cartilage as a landmark to find the cricoid— NOT as a location for pressure.

▶ The dominant thumb and forefinger should be used on the lateral borders of the cricoid ring.

Slide 2-27 **Cricoid Pressure Effects**

▶ Pressure is applied posteriorly for this maneuver, preventing higher pressures of air from ventilation techniques entering the esophagus, thus preventing regurgitation and aspiration of gastric contents.

▶ An adaptation of this maneuver may be used to assist those attempting to view the vocal cords during endotracheal intubation and should not be released until the cuff on the endotracheal tube is inflated.

Slide 2-28 **Continuous Positive Airway Pressure (CPAP)**

▶ Continuous positive airway pressure is positive pressure applied throughout the entire respiratory cycle via inspiratory and expiratory positive pressure.

▶ The patient must be spontaneously breathing with reliable ventilatory drive and adequate tidal volume.

▶ Indications:
— Ventilation support for those difficult to oxygenate because of conditions that reduce the functional residual capacity, such as congestive heart failure with pulmonary edema, atelectasis, or secretion retention
— Patients with airway edema or obstructive disease who need to maintain adequate ventilation
— Used in the hospital as a means of weaning patients from pressure support ventilators

▶ Non-invasive pressure support ventilation (NIPSV), also known as bilevel positive airway pressure (BiPAP) ventilation, is a noninvasive mode of ventilation in which there is a set level of both inspiratory and expiratory positive airway pressure. This may be applied through a nasal or full face mask.

Slide 2-29 **Medication-Assisted Intubation Introduction to RSI**

Slide 2-30 **Medication-Assisted Intubation (RSI) Procedures**

▶ Staged induction intubation (RSI) (This is not a rapid procedure!)

▶ Pose these two questions and provide support for pertinent answers prior to moving on.

Ask: *What procedures need to be completed in order to assure that this intubation will be successful?*

Ask: *What QA procedures should be in place in your system in order to prepare you for this procedure?*
— Performer knows limitations; has proven competency to medical director.
— Assesses the patient adequately for anatomic, physiologic contraindications to this technique.
— Has several backup plans in case the intubation cannot be performed once paralysis has been induced.

Slide 2-31 **The Steps to Successful RSI**

▶ Preparation: assessment, fall-back plans, monitors, IVs (two is best), supplies, equipment, position

SLIDE NO.   SLIDE TITLE/NOTES

▶ Pre-Oxygenation: (Provides an oxygen reservoir within the lungs. Washes out nitrogen, allowing for more apnea time.) 90–100% oxygen for at least 5 minutes. Try NOT to use BVM unless patient requires ventilation support prior to intubation (helps prevent aspiration).

▶ Pre-Treatment: With drugs used to minimize intubation side-effects:
— Lidocaine: For reactive airway disease and elevated ICP
— Opioid: To blunt sympathetic response
— Atropine: For children and relative bradycardia
— Defasciculation of Succinylcholine: For elevated ICP, high gastric pressures, eye injuries

▶ Paralysis with Induction: Sedative and paralytic—both short-acting, short half-life drugs

▶ Protection and Positioning: Sellick's maneuver, then position head/neck for intubation

▶ Placement and Proof: Intubate, inflate the cuff, then use two means of ETT confirmation.

▶ Post-Intubation Management: Secure ETT, ventilate, chest X-ray, end-tidal CO_2 or capnography, and monitor vital signs; long-term sedation and paralysis.

Slide 2-32 **Pre-RSI Anatomic Assessment**
▶ 3-3-2 Rule
— Anatomic assessment of the patient in an attempt to answer the question: Can I intubate this patient?
— Geometry of oral intubation: The first 3 of the 3-3-2 rule is three fingers between the teeth (can it open adequately?); the second 3 is measurement of the space from the mentum to the hyoid bone (diagram in previous slide) and identifies access to the airway. The 2 in the 3-3-2 rule requires two fingers be placed between the thyroid notch and the floor of the mandible. This identifies that the larynx is sufficiently low within the neck to permit oral access.

Slide 2-33 **Assess Before Acting . . .**
▶ Prior to giving medications . . .

Ask: *Can I intubate this patient?*
— An anatomic assessment should be performed (pre-RSI procedure).

Slide 2-34 **Mallampati Assessment, Pre-RSI**
▶ This identifies the amount of space available within the mouth for the insertion of both the laryngoscope and an ETT.
▶ The ideal patient position for this exam is a High Fowler's position with head in sniffing position and the patient sticking out his/her tongue.
▶ If the patient must be supine, use a tongue blade to mimic the tongue depression.

Slide 2-35 **The Lemon Law**
▶ Another mnemonic, LEMON, helps in assuring success in RSI.

NOTE: Mallampati assessment described on previous slide.

▸ Neck mobility: Attempt to take head/neck through range of motion (medical patient only), especially in the elderly. Patient places chin to chest, looks at the floor, then the ceiling.

Slide 2-36   **Pre-Treatment Drugs for RSI: LOAD**

▸ Review of drugs that may be given prior to sedation and paralysis (induction).

Slide 2-37   **General Procedures for RSI**

▸ Review the steps in medication-assisted intubation (RSI).

▸ Reinforce the length of time this procedures takes. ***This is not a rapid procedure!***

Slide 2-38   **SOAP ME Format—RSI Procedure**

▸ Another mnemonic for remembering the steps in RSI: SOAP ME as described on the slide.

▸ Reinforce that oxygen is added early so that nitrogen can be washed out.

Slide 2-39   **Failed Intubation Protocols**

▸ 99–100% of emergency department RSI procedures are successful because of the resources available as backup plans.

▸ The AHA cites a 50% failure rate amongst EMS systems with a low patient volume.

▸ Somewhere in between those two statistics for success rates in endotracheal intubation, the healthcare provider sees the need for backup plans if the intubation is not successful.

Ask: *Besides going "back to the basics," what are some procedures we can perform if the endotracheal tube is not properly inserted after giving sedatives and paralytics in a staged intubation attempt?*

▸ Support discussion:
— Combitube®, PtL® (remind them of the short-acting paralytic and use of dual-lumen, esophageal tubes)
— Supraglottic airways: King LT® or LMA®
— A second rescuer who is competent at intubating
— Digital intubation while patient is still paralyzed
— Cricothyrotomy (last resort)

Ask: *How long will the effects last for most sedatives/paralytics given in the initial induction?*

NOTE: Be patient here, allow for quick reference checks and book review with discussion.

Slide 2-40   **Failed Intubation Procedures**
Recap—provides some of the answers to first question on slide 2-39.

Slide 2-41   **Paralytic Duration of Action**
Recap—provides major answers to second question on slide 2-39.

Slide 2-42   **Scenario 1: The Unconscious Female**

▸ Have participants read the case on their own. Provide a synopsis of the information as it is displayed.

NOTES	SLIDE NO.	SLIDE TITLE/NOTES

Ask: *What does this scene tell you?*
- Scene size-up:
  — Entrance and exit available for your team?
  — Critical vs. non-critical situation?
  — Interpersonal dynamics?
- Stress that this patient is demonstrating "at risk" behavior, which places her at greater risk for communicable diseases.

NOTE: Do not move to the next slide until the answers are discussed.

Slide 2-43

Scenario 1: Initial Assessment
- General impression with ABCD perfusion. Have a participant read the information as you provide a synopsis.

Ask: *What would your initial treatment be?*
- Allow participants to discuss/provide potential answers.
  — Provide quick and simple airway positioning.
  — Suction.
  — Use pocket mask (with eventual oxygen) or BVM (with eventual oxygen) to immediately provide positive pressure ventilation. This will also help resuscitate the shock patient in bradycardia.
- Ask the related question below and discuss before moving on to the next slide.

Ask: *Should you treat the unstable patient or gather history?*
  — The unstable patient must have initial (basic) resuscitation prior to gathering history. (Review from Assessment/ Management lecture.)

Slide 2-44

Scenario 1
- Provides an outline of the answers to the previous slide's questions. Recap the initial assessment.

Slide 2-45

Additional Information
- Transition slide from the initial assessment to the SAMPLE history

Slide 2-46

Scenario 1
- Have participants read as you provide synopsis of information—reinforcing SAMPLE and OPQRST format.

Ask: *What does this information tell you?*
  — Unconsciousness is the chief complaint, therefore many of the history questions are not applicable.
- Read and discuss prior to asking next question.
  — Initial field impression
  — Differential impressions

Ask: *What part of the assessment should you do now?*
  — Focused physical exam
  — Possibly some OPQRST questions

Slide 2-47

Field Impression and Assessment
Recap—Provides an outline of the answers regarding the SAMPLE and OPQRST assessments.

Slide 2-48   **Focused Physical Examination**
▶ Have participants read as you provide synopsis of information—reinforcing the Focused Physical Exam and forming a field impression with differential diagnosis.

Ask: *What is your field impression? What other differential diagnoses could this be?*
▶ Discuss possible differential diagnoses.
▶ Have participants provide answers prior to asking next question.

Ask: *What would your initial treatment be?*
▶ Discuss prior to next slide.

Slide 2-49   **Field Impression and Differential Diagnosis**
Recap—Answers first question from slide 2-48.

Slide 2-50   **Immediate Plan of Care**
Recap—Answers second question from slide 2-48.

Slide 2-51   **Scenario 1**
▶ Have participants read the information, which you may also summarize.

Ask: *At what rate and depth should you ventilate this patient?*
▶ Discuss potential answers below prior to reading the next question.
▶ Demonstrate while counting so participants realize the "slow and low" ventilations that should be delivered.
— Rate of 10–12 per minute with inspiratory cycle over 1 second in patients with pulse; rate is 8–10 if no pulse.
— The ratio of inspiratory to expiratory time should be 1:2 (meaning that the inspiration should last 1 second and exhalation should occur over 2–3 seconds)

Ask: *What are some basic airway adjuncts that could be used for this patient?*
— Oropharyngeal airway
— Nasopharyngeal airway
— Esophageal tubes (PtL, DualLumen tube)
— Laryngeal airways
— Always have suction available

Slide 2-52   **Scenario 1**
▶ Review with participants.

Ask: *What are some advanced airway adjuncts that could be used?*
▶ Discuss prior to asking the next question on the slide.

Ask: *What are some of the contraindications to using the airway devices you have mentioned?*
▶ Discuss contraindications as participants provide the name of an acceptable advanced airway in this case.

Slide 2-53   **Scenario 1**
▶ Review the information so far: Patient gagged on an oral airway, has GCS of 5, is high risk for aspiration, and also needs to receive positive pressure ventilation.

NOTES	SLIDE NO.	SLIDE TITLE/NOTES

NOTE: In order to meet the objectives, tell the participants that the decision has been made to intubate.

Ask: *Does this patient need to be sedated prior to intubation?*

NOTE: Discuss first question prior to asking the second question on the slide.

▶ Take some time here. This can be controversial and participants will need guidance.

▶ Final answer depends on local protocols; one could argue that the patient has probably already been sedated.

▶ However, sedation in normal doses does not eliminate the gag reflex. The patient may bite down (reflexively) on the laryngoscope blade due to gag action.

Ask: *Will this patient need to receive a paralytic drug (along with sedation) prior to intubation?*

▶ Review indications for medication-assisted intubation, along with contraindications.

Slide 2-54

Scenario 1

▶ To meet objective, first discuss medication-assisted intubation with sedation only.

Ask: *What might you expect with sedation only for side effects/complications?*
— Tight airway due to intact gag reflex
— Side effects from the sedative used (see PDR)

Ask: *What should we do now?*
▶ Allow for guided discussion prior to the next slide.

Slide 2-55

Options

Recap procedures used when sedation only does not allow for successful intubation.

Slide 2-56

Scenario 1

▶ Review update information with participants.
▶ Review depth of placement procedures for ETT.

Ask: *What cm marking should be at the patient's lip?*
— Generally 3 times the tube size (± 1), 21 for females and 24 for slides

Ask: *What confirmation procedures should be used for ETT placement?*
— 3–5 point auscultation
— End-tidal CO_2 detection (colormetric, capnography)
— Esophageal detector device

Slide 2-57

Intubation Assessment Devices

Recap of answer to question 2 on slide 2-56.

▶ Esophageal tube check: Creates a suction force at the tracheal (distal) end of the ETT, either by pulling back on a plunger of a syringe or compressing a bulb. It is based on the ability to readily aspirate air from the cartilage-supported trachea by drawing from gas in the lower airways.
— Not reliable in patients younger than 4–5 years of age, who are morbidly obese, or in late pregnancy.

SLIDE NO.	SLIDE TITLE/NOTES	NOTES

► Exhaled or end-tidal CO_2 monitoring: a colormetric device attached between the positioned ETT and the positive pressure ventilation device.
— Ventilate patient at a normal rate for 6 cycles before assessing the true color of the device.
  ▪ Yellow indicates CO_2 is being detected—the ETT should be in the trachea.
  ▪ Tan means that there may be poor blood flow to the lungs.
— Ventilate six more times and recheck color; find the cause for poor lung perfusion (PE, arrest).
  ▪ If the color remains purple in a patient with a pulse (good perfusion), the ETT is probably in the esophagus. The color should change from purple to yellow with *each* breath (not stay yellow). If the patient's lungs are receiving poor or no blood flow, this device may be unreliable.

Slide 2-58 **Scenario 1**
► Remind participants of the status of this case. The patient has been successfully intubated and position has been assured via two methods.
► Ask and discuss this question before showing and discussing the second question on the slide.

Ask: *What rate and tidal volume should we ventilate this patient?*
— "Slow and low" is advocated. A rate of about 10–12 per minute with a tidal volume that just barely allows the chest to rise slowly, over 1 second. Normal lungs are usually set at an inspiratory/expiratory ratio of 1:2.

NOTE: It is sometimes helpful to demonstrate with your hands (mimick holding a BVM) the 1 second duration. Inspiratory time at a ratio of 1:2 at a rate of 10–12 per minute.

Ask: *If monitoring patient's CO_2 levels, what measurement is ideal?*
— Continuous capnography measurements (if available) should show a normal level (35–45 mmHg) unless specifically directed by medical direction.

Slide 2-59 **Ventilation Considerations**
Recap of answers to questions on previous slide.

NOTE: You may need to explain "herniation syndrome" as it applies to increasing ICP. This procedure for hyperventilation is protocol driven and specific to finding Cushing's reflex with pupil changes—and is thought of as a resuscitation to prevent herniation of the brain through the foramen magnum. Allowing the CO_2 levels to fall below 35 for an extended period of time dramatically decreases blood flow to the brain.
► Provide summary of Scenario 1.

Slide 2-60 **Scenario 2**
► Present if time allows.

SLIDE NO.	SLIDE TITLE/NOTES
Slide 2-61	**Scenario 2: Scene Size-up** ▶ Provide a synopsis of this case as participants read it. This is a postcode patient who is being ventilated via ETT.
Slide 2-62	**Scenario 2** **Ask:** *What complication could be occurring?* ▶ Discuss answers to this question prior to viewing and discussing the next question on this slide. **Ask:** *What complications occur suddenly in the intubated patient?* **Ask:** *What actions should be taken to correct this problem?* ▶ As participants offer answers to question 1, go back and ask what they would do to correct it. ▶ Reinforce the need for securing ETT and routine reassessment for depth of placement (cm mark at the lip) because simple head/torso movement can completely dislodge an ETT.
Slide 2-63	**Complication in the Intubated Patient** ▶ This mnemonic, DOPE, is taken from the AHA's PALS course. — It is a quick way to remember what can go wrong in an intubated patient.
Slide 2-64	**Scenario 2** **Ask:** *What should be done to correct the problem?*
Slide 2-65	**Complications in the Intubated Patient** ▶ Review the sudden and severe complications that may occur in the intubated patient. Review procedures to correct the problem.
Slide 2-66	**Summary** End of Scenario 2.
Slide 2-67	**References** ▶ The instructor should point out certain websites for some of the newer airway devices.

⊞ CHAPTER 4: HYPOPERFUSION (SHOCK)

SLIDE   **SLIDE TITLE/NOTES**

Slide 4-1   **Hypoperfusion**
Introduction

Slide 4-2   **Physiological Changes in Response to Shock**
▶ Discuss the physiological changes that occur in response to shock.
▶ As cardiac output drops (for whatever reason), baroreceptors in the arch of the aorta sense the change and stimulate the systemic response:
— Sympathetic nervous system stimulates the adrenal medullae to secrete catecholamines.
— Catecholamines stimulate alpha and beta receptors sites in heart, lungs, blood vessels, and sweat glands to cause:
▪ vasoconstriction
▪ bronchodilation
▪ increased heart rate
▪ increased cardiac contraction
▶ As decreased oxygen and glucose supplies to cells continue:
— Kidneys sense a drop in pressure and release renin.
— Renin stimulates the production of Angiotensin I.
— Angiotensin I is converted to Angiotensin II, which is a powerful vasoconstrictor.
— Angiotensin II stimulates the production of aldosterone, which acts on the kidney to conserve water.

Slide 4-3   **Alpha and Beta Receptor Site Activity Within Sympathetic Nervous System**
▶ Review the determinates of BP (CO × PVR) and their relationship to alpha stimulation.
▶ Illustrate to participants the ease of using the CARDIO mnemonic in remembering beta properties.
▶ Relate these activities to the signs and symptoms of shock.

Slide 4-4   **Cell Death in Shock**
▶ Walk participants through the steps to cell death in shock; discuss what happens in each step.
— Shift from aerobic to anaerobic metabolism
— Failure of Na^+-ATP pump with intracellular accumulation of Na^+
— Intracellular swelling including cellular mitochondria, resulting in further loss of cellular energy sources
— Breakdown of lysosomes with cellular destruction and death
▶ Remind participants that a collection of like cells make up tissues, like tissues make up organs and like organs make up systems. As more and more cells die, so do tissues, organs, and then systems.

Slide 4-5   **Factors in the Severity of Shock**
▶ Type of shock: Anaphylactic shock may appear within minutes whereas septic shock may take days to appear.

- Age of patient: In younger patients, it takes less to induce shock. In older patients, the compensatory mechanisms may take longer to begin response.
- Pre-existing disorders: Compensatory mechanism may be malfunctioning or not functioning at all.
- Speed of onset: The slower the onset, the more time for the patient to compensate.
- Effects of drugs and other substances: Drugs such as beta blockers, ACE inhibitors, and others may block portions of the compensatory response. Alcohol and other recreation drugs can interfere with the body's normal response to shock, or even result in neurogenic shock.

Slide 4-6   A Review of the Four Major Types of Shock

- It is essential that the organs or systems be reviewed to identify the cause of shock so that the appropriate treatment can be initiated.

Slide 4-7   Hemorrhagic Shock

- Compensated (early) hemorrhagic shock signs and symptoms. You may want to relate these (again) to the pathophysiology of shock discussed earlier in this presentation.

Slide 4-8   Progressive Hemorrhagic Shock

- Compensation mechanisms begin to recede as blood loss continues in hemorrhagic shock—related to these signs and symptoms.

NOTE: The symptoms displayed here should be related to the previously discussed pathophysiology and response in shock.

- Point out that BP begins to fall in this phase.

NOTE: Classic shock signs should be a review for participants.

Slide 4-9   Irreversible Hemorrhagic Shock

- Irreversible shock signs and symptoms in hemorrhagic shock reflect the circulation of acids, enzymes, microemboli with cell damage, and death . . . organ failure.
- Tell participants they will now compare the signs and symptoms of hemorrhagic shock (previously taught as classic shock) to those of anaphylactic shock.

Slide 4-10   Comparison of Anaphylactic to Hemorrhagic Shock

- State that there are many different agents that can cause an anaphylactic reaction.
- Route of exposure can be via injection, ingestion, absorption, or inhalation.
- Anaphylactic shock is a form of distributive shock.
- Emphasize that it is an exaggerated immune response that along with a distributive shock causes angioedema to the airway.
- Mast cells release histamine, SRSA (slow reacting substance of anaphylaxis), heparin, platelet-activating factors, and other chemicals that cause widespread vasodilation and blood vessel leaking (flushed skin with hives, petechiae, and itching).

▶ Vessel permeability also causes widespread edema, especially in the mucous membranes (wheezing, stridor, rales).

▶ Smooth muscle contraction in GI tract may result in cramping, vomiting, and diarrhea.

▶ Profound hypotension with dyspnea is a common presentation.

▶ Discuss the onset of signs and severity of reaction.

— Speed of the reaction depends on the degree of sensitivity the patient has previously developed, route of exposure, and the target organ.

— Healthcare provider can anticipate that if time of exposure and onset of symptoms are close together, the overall reaction will be severe.

— Determining the difference between mild and severe anaphylaxis governs the treatment.

Slide 4-11   Hypovolemic Shock vs. Hemorrhagic Shock

Ask: *What types of medical conditions can present with non-hemorrhagic hypovolemic shock?*

— Nonketotic hyperosmolar syndrome

— DKA

— Gastrointestinal losses

— Third spacing

▶ Review the physiologic changes of aging and signs of shock.

NOTE: Segue into next slide by stating that there are four categories of shock; let's look at obstructive shock next.

Slide 4-12   Obstructive Shock

▶ Describe the pathophysiology behind the inability of the myocardium to adequately fill due to the pressure exerted on it or the blockages preventing the flow of blood—interference with preload and afterload.

▶ Cardiac tamponade causes inadequate filling pressure of the heart.

▶ Pulmonary embolism and tension pneumothorax result in inadequate venous return to the heart.

Slide 4-13   Pulmonary Embolus

Ask: *What conditions increase the risk of pulmonary embolism?*

— Obesity

— Recent immobility or recent surgery

— Patient taking oral contraceptives, especially among smokers

— Hereditary coagulation disorders

▶ Pulmonary embolus interferes with preload to the left ventricle.

▶ Chest pain is not always present—if it is, it is usually pleuritic in nature. Lung sounds are usually clear.

▶ Certain clot showers may create syncope and cardiac arrest, arrhythmias like PVCs, and atrial fibrillation.

▶ Treatment is generally supportive in the prehospital setting.

Slide 4-14   Cardiac Tamponade

▶ Point out that tamponade is usually associated with a trauma etiology.

Ask: *What medical conditions can cause a pericardial tamponade?*
  — Pericardial effusion (inflammatory, infectious, neoplastic)
  — Rare outside of trauma
▶ Pericardial tamponade restricts cardiac filling.
▶ May present with a paradoxical pulse with hypoxia.
▶ Beck's Triad is the classic presentation: narrowed pulse pressure, distended neck veins, and distant heart sounds.
▶ Point out the difficulties inherent in assessing for Beck's Triad in the field.
▶ Point out the major clinical differentiation of diminished breath sounds in tension pneumothorax vs. tamponade.

NOTE: Whether prehospital personnel can perform pericardiocentesis or not, it is important for the provider to identify and report these symptoms and the history that supports the development of this condition.

Slide 4-15   Tension Pneumothorax

Ask: *What medical conditions can lead to a tension pneumothorax?*
  — COPD—ruptured bleb
  — Over-inflation injuries
▶ The most common cause of pneumothorax is a mechanically ventilated patient.
▶ Differentiate between signs and symptoms of a simple pneumothorax, tension pneumothorax, and pericardial tamponade.
▶ Positive pressure ventilation should not be withheld from patients with a tension pneumothorax, but the provider must understand that the condition may worsen.
▶ Definitive treatment is needle decompression.
▶ Review the correct procedure for this critical treatment.

NOTE: Segue to the next slide, which reviews the next type of shock, distributive, which was partially covered in the first case study.

Slide 4-16   Distributive Shock
▶ The problem is not a decreased volume or obstructed flow of blood, but rather an extreme vasodilation and increased capillary permeability, causing a relative hypovolemia.
▶ Not enough fluid to fill the larger tank.

Slide 4-17   Neurogenic Shock

Ask: *What medical conditions can result in neurogenic shock?*
  — Toxins from infections and poisons
  — Extreme parasympathetic discharge from an overdose
  — Association with traumatic injury to the spinal column or spinal cord
▶ Widespread vasodilation is usually due to loss of sympathetic response. The signs and symptoms differ from "classic" shock because of this pathophysiology. Skin vitals do not fit the picture! Heart rate does not fit the picture!
▶ Pulmonary edema may occur with drug- or poison-induced shock along with severe compromise in respirations.

(Discuss how a narcotic overdose results in pinpoint pupils compared with cerebral hypoxia, in which the patient develops dilated pupils.)

▶ Treatment is aimed at supporting the dilated vessels and administration of an antidote. Follow local protocols for antidote but naloxone, glucagon, or flumazenil may be considered. If lungs are clear, controlled fluid boluses may be considered until vasopressors may be administered.

Slide 4-18   **Septic Shock**

▶ Result of an overwhelming infection. *Altered mental status is the key sign/symptom if there is a history of illness/infection or fever.*

▶ Release of bacterial or viral toxins that cause vasodilation and increased permeability.

▶ Discuss potential causes, such as:
— Respiratory infections
— Decubitus ulcers
— Urinary tract infections

▶ There may be a wide variety of symptoms, depending on the organism, strength of the patient's immune system, inflammatory response, and the involved tissues/organs. First stage is hypermetabolism; last stage is shock.

▶ The very young and very old may not present with fever.

▶ DO NOT confuse the symptoms of dyspnea with changes in lung sounds with CHF.

▶ Multi-system organ dysfunction many times is the result of this type of shock with widespread microemboli.

▶ Treatment is aimed at early antibiotic coverage with vessel support, with first judicious fluid administration and vasopressor drugs.

NOTE: Segue to the next slide on cardiogenic shock.

Slide 4-19   **Cardiogenic Shock**

Ask: *What are the causes of cardiogenic shock besides an AMI?*
— Valvular insufficiency
— Rhythm disturbances

▶ If caused by an AMI, then a large part of the myocardium will be damaged or stunned.

Slide 4-20   **Cardiogenic Shock vs. Hemorrhagic**

▶ Emphasize the differences between cardiogenic and hypovolemic shock.
— You must be able to differentiate the two because the treatment of each can be fatal if employed for the wrong pathophysiological condition.
— Aggressive fluid therapy can be fatal in the presence of cardiogenic shock, and vasopressors can be harmful if inadequate fluid resuscitation is present in hypovolemic shock. Emphasize the findings of orthopnea and PND.

▶ Review the standards in pharmacologic management of cardiogenic shock, according to ACLS guidelines.

SLIDE NO.	SLIDE TITLE/NOTES

NOTE: Segue to next slide by introducing Scenario 1.

Slide 4-21   **Scenario 1: Scene Size-up**
- ▶ Have participants read the case study to themselves. Then provide a synopsis as the slide appears.

Ask: *What is the scene telling you?*
— The problem is probably medical.
— There is one patient.
— This appears to be a safe medical scene so far.
— No need for additional resources at this time.

Ask: *What is the patient telling you?*
— He is in respiratory distress and is potentially unstable.
— He had recent surgery or injury to his foot.
— He is older and possibly may have complicating medical conditions.

Slide 4-22   **Scenario 1: Initial Assessment**
- ▶ Have participants read the case study to themselves. Then provide a synopsis as the slide appears.
- ▶ Initial assessment: Look for life threats and intervene if necessary.
- ▶ Initial impression:
  — He is in distress.
  — He is in respiratory distress.
  — He is showing signs and symptoms of hypoperfusion.
  — He is unstable.
- ▶ Point out that when looking for an initial impression you can also ask:
  — What may be wrong with this patient?
  — What else could be wrong?
  — What should be done next?
- ▶ This could be a GI bleed; ruptured bowel, appendix, or other structure; sepsis; sickle cell crisis; food poisoning; etc.
- ▶ Oxygen, IVs, and considering early transport may also be presented.

Slide 4-23   **Scenario 1: OPQRST History**
- ▶ Point out several items in this history. The healthcare provider used the classic 1–10 (or 0–10) scale in the description of severity of dyspnea.
  - O Fairly rapid onset.
  - P Sitting up relieves respiratory distress.
  - Q Vague discomfort: "jumping out of my skin"—suggests skin involvement.
  - R Does not apply.
  - S Dyspnea is severe.
  - T Condition is worsening. Syncope suggests hypoperfusion.
- ▶ Initial impression: shock, possible AMI with failure, sepsis, anaphylaxis.

Slide 4-24   **Scenario 1: SAMPLE History**
- ▶ Ask for the participants' field impressions. Then tie into the participants' list of what may be wrong with the

patient a list of differential diagnoses that need to be ruled in/out.

▶ Review the following:

S   Suggests a respiratory problem such as sepsis and anaphylaxis.

A   None—tends to rule out anaphylaxis—unless this is the first time for this allergic reaction.

M   Vasotec and Motrin: The Vasotec is an ACE inhibitor and could inhibit the patient's BP response, or cause hypotension if taken with alcohol. It may also cause angioedema of the upper airway. Motrin is associated with GI bleeds and allergic reactions.

P   Hypertension: Check the patient's normal blood pressure 140/90 on medication. His foot bunionectomy 2 days ago suggests the patient has been immobile; therefore, a pulmonary emboli should also be suspected.

L   The patient has eaten, but a blood sugar check may still be indicated.

E   Because he is older, you should evaluate for an AMI. His food intake should be evaluated for possible allergic response.

Slide 4-25   Scenario 1: Focused Assessment

▶ Relate this additional information to the participants to reinforce their field impression.

▶ In order to better understand, compare the signs and symptoms of anaphylactic shock to the other types of shock (or classic signs/symptoms).

— This patient is probably suffering from anaphylactic shock due to the hives and bilateral wheezing.

— Hemorrhagic shock tends to present with cool, pale, diaphoretic skin and clear lungs.

— Septic shock may involve the lungs, but skin is not blotchy with hives, so sepsis is probably ruled out.

— Pulmonary emboli may cause shock, but once again does not usually present with blotchy skin and hives or wheezes.

Slide 4-26   General Management of Shock

▶ Discuss the general principles of shock management.

NOTE: This slide reinforces why it is important for the provider to determine the target organ—differential for the type of shock in the assessment because management is centered around the mechanism.

▶ Giving large amounts of crystalloids is of limited benefit in anaphylaxis.

▶ Treatment needs to be focused on limiting the allergic/immune response with pharmacologic agents.

Slide 4-27   Scenario 1: Differential Diagnosis

▶ Point out that determining the cause of the shock is integral in providing the correct management. Initial impression with differential diagnosis begins with a thorough history and physical exam.

▶ Types of shock are known either by the primary organ of dysfunction or by the primary cause of dysfunction. History will determine which symptoms began to appear first, possibly indicating which organ is primary.

Slide 4-28   **Specific Management of Anaphylactic Shock**
▶ Controlled fluid administration to challenge preload of the heart and begin to replace fluids lost due to third spacing.
▶ If wheezing with hypotension, a bronchodilator is indicated but with caution in patients with severe cardiovascular effects.
▶ Epinephrine is indicated in allergic reaction due to its alpha and beta stimulation, along with its ability to limit histamine release from the mast cell.
▶ This drug can be given SC or IV, but IV dose is usually reserved for severe cardiovascular collapse. *Ranitidine, famotidine, and cimetidine can be adjuncts to control urticaria and severe reactions. Dopamine should be considered for persistent hypotension.*

NOTE: Epinephrine should be used with caution in patients older than 40 with cardiac history because it increases myocardial oxygen demands.

Slide 4-29   **Scenario 1: Additional Information**
▶ Some controlled fluid boluses may be administered to replace that lost due to third spacing.
▶ If a patient presents with a mild case of allergic reaction, epinephrine may not be necessary. Diphenhydramine (Benadryl), a potent antihistamine, can be administered either IV or IM for relief of minor reactions. *Steroids can be considered for field treatment of allergic reactions, but effects occur hours later. Glucagon is considered for patients taking beta blockers who do not respond to epinephrine.*

Slide 4-30   **Scenario 1: Follow-Up**
Follow-up for Case Study 1

Slide 4-31   **Scenario 2**
▶ You may provide a synopsis of this information after the participants read it to themselves.

Ask: *What is the scene telling you?*
— The problem is probably medical, but trauma cannot be ruled out.
— There is one patient.
— This appears to be a safe scene so far.
— No need for additional resources at this time.

Ask: *What is the patient telling you?*
— He is in respiratory distress and is potentially unstable.
— He is older and possibly may have complicating medical conditions.
— This condition is worse than his normal condition.

Slide 4-32 **Scenario 2: Initial Assessment**
- ▶ Provide a synopsis and then. . . .

Ask: *What treatment needs to be instituted before we move on?*
- — Initial assessment: Look for life threats and intervene if necessary.
- — Initial impression:
  - ▪ He is in distress.
  - ▪ He is in respiratory distress.
  - ▪ He is showing signs and symptoms of hypoperfusion.
  - ▪ He is not mentating well.
  - ▪ He is unstable.
- ▶ Point out that when looking for an initial impression you can also ask:
- — What may be wrong with this patient?
- — What else could be wrong?
- — What should be done next?
- ▶ This could be an AMI, CHF, COPD, pulmonary emboli, sepsis, or pneumonia.
- ▶ Oxygen, monitor, IVs, and considering early transport may also be presented.

Slide 4-33 **Scenario 2: Initial Treatment**
- ▶ Review information then ask and discuss the following, one at a time:
- — What assessment(s) need to be done next?
- — What history needs to be acquired?

Slide 4-34 **Scenario 2: OPQRST History**
- ▶ Give an overview of the information.

Ask: *What is your field impression?*
- — This could be an AMI, CHF, COPD, pulmonary emboli, sepsis, pneumonia, or GI bleed.
- ▶ Provide positive reinforcement and compile the list of possibilities as differential diagnoses that need to be ruled in/out.
- O Gradual onset.
- P Suggests hypovolemic cause to the hypoperfusion.
- Q Suggest a possible respiratory, cardiac, or GI problem.
- R Does not rule out any possibilities.
- S The pain is not severe, but the elderly may not have good pain perception.
- T Suggests a chronic condition causing his pain.

Slide 4-35 **Scenario 2: SAMPLE History**
- ▶ Review this information and revisit the list of differential diagnoses.

Ask: *Have any impressions from the previous list been ruled out/in with this information?*
- S Suggests an infectious process.
- A Decreases any suspicion of anaphylaxis.
- M Metformin (Glucophage) is an oral anti-hyperglycemic agent that may cause lactic acidosis. Hypotension, nausea, and vomiting may occur if ingested with alcohol.

Captopril (Capoten), an ACE inhibitor, may cause hypotension if ingested with alcohol, and is associated with angioedema. Atenolol (Tenormin) is a beta blocker and may not allow normal increases in heart rate and BP to compensate for shock. ASA (aspirin) may be associated with a GI bleed.

P Diabetes indicates a need to evaluate the blood sugar and possible decreased pain perception; he has a positive cardiac history and should be evaluated for an AMI or CHF. He may have more adhesions and a possible bowel obstruction or his cancer has returned.

L Suggests GI, concern for blood sugar.

E Hypovolemia.

Slide 4-36   **Scenario 2: Focused Assessment**

▶ Review this information.

Ask: *What type of shock might this be?*

— Vital signs suggest septic shock. Drains increase the potential for infection and sepsis along with history of two days illness and fever.

▶ Review the major signs and symptoms with history and findings on physical exam.

▶ Review the prehospital treatment needed for urosepsis and shock.

Slide 4-37   **Scenario 2: Additional Information**

▶ Review this information and then ask participants what treatment they recommend. Additional management should include determining the blood glucose level and 12 lead EKG monitoring.

Slide 4-38   **Scenario 2: Follow-Up Information**

▶ The participants have been ordered to provide a dopamine infusion to this septic shock patient after fluid bolus, oxygen, and monitors.

▶ Have participants discuss how to calculate this infusion with the parameters given on the slide. (Slide 4-39 provides the answer.)

OPTION: Have a volunteer go to a board and provide the math for this.

Slide 4-39   **Scenario 2: Dopamine Infusion Calculation**

▶ Brief overview of calculation

— Calculate the dose desired by multiplying patient's weight in kilograms by the amount of micrograms per minute ordered ($80 \times 10 = 800$)

— Calculate the dose available by converting the drug supplied (400 mg) into micrograms (400,000) and instilling it into the solution of 500 ml.

— Calculate how many micrograms in each ml.

$$\frac{\text{Dose Desired}}{\text{Dose Available}} \times \text{Drip Set} = \text{Drops Per Minute}$$

SLIDE NO.	SLIDE TITLE/NOTES	NOTES

Slide 4-40   **Scenario 2: Follow-Up**
Presents follow-up of Scenario 2.

Slide 4-41   **Summary/Overview—Treatment in Shock**
Emphasize individual treatments for each type of shock.

Slide 4-42   **Summary/Overview—Treatment in Shock (continued)**
Emphasize individual treatments for each type of shock.

Slide 4-43   **Summary Slide for Hypoperfusion Presentation in AMLS**
The healthcare provider must learn to suspect shock, conduct a thorough assessment, recognize the target organ affected and then the type of shock, and provide the specific management needed.

CHAPTER 5: DYSPNEA, RESPIRATORY DISTRESS, OR RESPIRATORY FAILURE

SLIDE NO.	SLIDE TITLE/NOTES

Slide 5-1

Introduction

Dyspnea, Respiratory Distress, or Respiratory Failure
▶ Ask participants to give their definition of dyspnea.
▶ Dyspnea is one of the more complex differentials to make, because so many etiologies can have shortness of breath as a sign or symptom.

Slide 5-2

Introduction
▶ Discuss the frequency of this type of call.
▶ Discuss the many presentations of a dyspnea call from someone who is afraid that patient has no danger of life threat, but will die soon if action is not taken immediately.
▶ Emphasize the potential for a life-threatening emergency.

Slide 5-3

Anatomy and Physiology
▶ Review how the structures work together to deliver oxygen to the alveoli and to remove carbon dioxide.
▶ Differentiate between the upper and lower airways.
▶ The larynx is usually the dividing point between the upper and lower airways. Remind participants that it is useful to determine if a problem is in the upper or the lower airway.
▶ Discuss respiratory patterns as well and their implications.

Slide 5-4

Anatomy and Physiology (continued)

Ask: *Where do you assess for breath sounds?*
— Breath sounds should be assessed bilaterally, contrasted from side to side, at the axilla and at the back.
— Discuss various breath sounds and their implications.

Slide 5-5

Minute Volume
▶ Minute volume is the volume of air exchanged in the lungs in one minute. It is critical to evaluate the rate and depth of ventilations. Even though you may not have an exact measurement, the principle of minute volume still applies.
▶ Examples of minute volume:
Ventilatory Rate × Tidal Volume = Minute Volume
12 × 500 cc = 6000 cc
12 × 200 cc = 2400 cc
— The patient is breathing, but the minute volume is inadequate because he is breathing too shallow.
30 × 200 cc = 6000 cc
— The patient is breathing, the minute volume is adequate, but the rate is fast. The work of breathing to maintain an adequate tidal volume has increased.

Ask: *How can you identify increased work of breathing?*

Slide 5-6

Muscles of Respiration
▶ Review with participants that accessory muscle use is an indicator of increased work of breathing.

▶ There are both external and internal intercostal muscles that can be used to increase ventilatory flow when the patient is in distress.

Slide 5-7   **Important to Note . . .**

▶ Emphasize not using PaO_2 or O_2 saturations as the determining factor. Look at the patient's work of breathing and accessory muscle use. A patient who is laboring to breathe needs intervention regardless of PaO_2 levels.

▶ Transition to the next slide with the following question.

Ask: *Besides use of accessory muscles, what other indicators may be present at the scene to suggest a respiratory problem?*

— Home oxygen devices, medication, piles or bags of tissues, etc.

Slide 5-8   **Scene Size-up**

▶ Follow up answer to previous question. Summarize responses and add any of these the participants did not verbalize.

Slide 5-9   **Assessing Respiratory Compromise**

▶ Review and caution participants about bradypnea and impending respiratory arrest.

Slide 5-10   **Important to Note . . .**

▶ Emphasize aggressive airway management and ventilation in the presence of respiratory failure.

Slide 5-11   **Scenario 1: Scene Size-up**

▶ Allow participants to call out their responses.

▶ Reinforce: Location, potential for exposure to environment, toxins, bites, stings, age of patient, and types of problems to anticipate.

▶ The scene is safe.

▶ Summarize by reporting that the initial assessment indicates a potentially critical patient.

Slide 5-12   **Scenario 1—Initial Assessment**

▶ Discuss any factors not brought out in the previous slide. Reinforce chronic vs. acute, potential for multiple problems, and the need for additional assessment, which transitions to the next slide.

▶ Discuss initial management to include oxygen and possible nebulized albuterol, and removal from environment.

Slide 5-13   **Scenario 1—Focused History**

▶ Discuss the findings and potential differential/field diagnoses.

Slide 5-14   **Scenario 1—Focused History**

▶ Discuss the findings.

Slide 5-15   **Scenario 1—Focused Physical Exam**

▶ Discuss the findings and generate differential field diagnoses.

Slide 5-16   **Scenario 1—Discussion**

▶ Discuss the potential differential field diagnoses and the process (pertinent negatives, rule outs, physical findings, onset) they used to come to the diagnosis.

Slide 5-17   **Scenario 1—Field Diagnosis and Treatment Options**
- Discuss the treatment options. Acknowledge variances for local protocols.
- Emphasize that epinephrine is the essential and most important treatment, and that is the only treatment that really reverses the anaphylaxis process acutely.
- Bronchodilators have an immediate effect also, but do not attack the underlying pathophysiology. H1 and H2 blockers are helpful primarily for itching and urticaria, and corticosteroids have a delayed effect. IV fluid for those with hypotension due to vasodilatation is helpful.

Slide 5-18   **Scenario 2—Scene Size-up**
- Review the list. Include any answers not addressed.
- Allow participants to call out their responses.
- Reinforce: Location, age, recent activity, color, appearance.
- The scene is safe.
- Summarize by reporting that the initial assessment indicates a potentially critical patient.

Slide 5-19   **Scenario 2—Initial Assessment**
- Discuss any factors not brought out in the previous slide. Reinforce chronic vs. acute, potential for multiple problems, and the need for additional assessment, which transitions to the next slide.
- Discuss initial management to include oxygen and possible nebulized albuterol and a cardiac evaluation.

Slide 5-20   **Scenario 2—Focused History**
- As you progress through the causes of dyspnea, relate them to the case study.
- Discuss the findings and potential differential/field diagnoses.

Slide 5-21   **Scenario 2—Focused History**
- Discuss the findings.

Slide 5-22   **Scenario 2—Focused Physical Exam**
- Have participants discuss and justify. They do not all have to agree with each other.
- Discuss the findings and generate differential field diagnoses.

Slide 5-23   **Scenario 2—Discussion**
- Discuss the potential differential field diagnoses and the process (pertinent negatives, rule outs, physical findings, onset) they used to come to the diagnosis.

Slide 5-24   **Scenario 2—Field Diagnosis and Treatment Options**
- Discuss the treatment options. Acknowledge variances for local protocols.
- Typical pneumococcal pneumonia presents with a fairly acute development of fever, rusty sputum, and shortness of breath.

Slide 5-25   **Scenario 3—Scene Size-up**
- Reinforce: Location, age, recent activity, color, appearance.
- The scene is safe.
- Summarize by reporting that the initial assessment indicates a potentially critical patient.

SLIDE NO.	SLIDE TITLE/NOTES	NOTES

Slide 5-26 **Scenario 3—Initial Assessment**
- ▶ Discuss any factors not brought out in the previous slide. Reinforce chronic vs. acute, potential for multiple problems, and the need for additional assessment, which transitions to the next slide.
- ▶ Discuss initial management to include oxygen, IV fluids, and further assessment.

Slide 5-27 **Scenario 3—Focused History**
- ▶ Discuss the findings and potential differential/field diagnoses.

Slide 5-28 **Scenario 3—Focused History**
- ▶ Discuss the findings.

Slide 5-29 **Scenario 3—Focused Physical Exam**
- ▶ Discuss the findings and generate differential field diagnoses.

Slide 5-30 **Scenario 3—Discussion**
- ▶ Discuss the potential differential field diagnoses and the process (pertinent negatives, rule outs, physical findings, onset) they used to come to the diagnosis.

Slide 5-31 **Scenario 3—Field Diagnosis and Treatment Options**
- ▶ Discuss the treatment options. Acknowledge variances for local protocols.

Slide 5-32 **Scenario 4—Scene Size-up**
- ▶ Allow participants to call out their responses.
- ▶ Reinforce: Location, age, recent activity, color, appearance.
- ▶ The scene is safe.
- ▶ Summarize by reporting that the initial assessment indicates a potentially critical patient.

Slide 5-33 **Scenario 4—Initial Assessment**
- ▶ Discuss any factors not brought out in the previous slide.
- ▶ Reinforce chronic vs. acute, potential for multiple problems, and the need for additional assessment, which transitions to the next slide.
- ▶ Discuss initial management to include suctioning, position to facilitate airway support, oxygen and possible fluid challenge, and a cardiac evaluation.

Slide 5-34 **Scenario 4—Focused History**
- ▶ Discuss the findings and potential differential/field diagnoses.

Slide 5-35 **Scenario 4—Focused History**
- ▶ Discuss the findings.

Slide 5-36 **Scenario 4—Focused Physical Exam**
- ▶ Discuss the findings and generate differential field diagnoses.

Slide 5-37 **Scenario 4—Discussion**
- ▶ Discuss the potential differential field diagnoses and the process (pertinent negatives, rule outs, physical findings, onset) they used to come to the diagnosis.

Slide 5-38 **Scenario 4—Field Diagnosis and Treatment Options**
- ▶ Discuss the treatment options. Acknowledge variances for local protocols.

SLIDE NO.	SLIDE TITLE/NOTES
Slide 5-39	**Scenario 5—Scene Size-up** ▶ Allow participants to call out their responses. ▶ Reinforce: Location, age, recent activity, color, appearance. ▶ The scene is safe. ▶ Summarize by reporting that the initial assessment indicates a potentially critical patient.
Slide 5-40	**Scenario 5—Initial Assessment** ▶ Discuss any factors not brought out in the previous slide. ▶ Reinforce chronic vs. acute, potential for multiple problems, and the need for additional assessment, which transitions to the next slide. ▶ Discuss initial management to include high flow oxygen and IV therapy.
Slide 5-41	**Scenario 5—Focused History** ▶ Discuss the findings and potential differential/field diagnoses.
Slide 5-42	**Scenario 5—Focused History** ▶ Discuss the findings.
Slide 5-43	**Scenario 5—Focused Physical Exam** ▶ Discuss the findings and generate differential field diagnoses. Discuss chronic vs. acute presentation.
Slide 5-44	**Scenario 5—Discussion** ▶ Discuss the potential differential field diagnoses and the process (pertinent negatives, rule outs, physical findings, onset) they used to come to the diagnosis.
Slide 5-45	**Scenario 5—Field Diagnosis and Treatment Options** ▶ Discuss the potential differential field diagnoses and the process (pertinent negatives, rule outs, physical findings, onset) they used to come to the diagnosis.
Slide 5-46	**Scenario 6—Scene Size-up** ▶ Allow participants to call out their responses. ▶ Reinforce: Location, age, recent activity, color, appearance. ▶ The scene is safe. ▶ Summarize by reporting that the initial assessment indicates a potentially critical patient.
Slide 5-47	**Scenario 6—Initial Assessment** ▶ Discuss any factors not brought out in the previous slide. ▶ Reinforce chronic vs. acute, potential for multiple problems, and the need for additional assessment, which transitions to the next slide. ▶ Discuss initial management to include oxygen and IV therapy.
Slide 5-48	**Scenario 6—Focused History** ▶ Discuss the findings and potential differential/field diagnoses.
Slide 5-49	**Scenario 6—Focused History** ▶ Discuss the findings.

Slide 5-50   **Scenario 6—Focused Physical Exam**
- ▶ Discuss the findings and generate differential field diagnoses. Discuss chronic vs. acute presentation.

Slide 5-51   **Scenario 6—Discussion**
- ▶ Discuss the potential differential field diagnoses and the process (pertinent negatives, rule outs, physical findings, onset) they used to come to the diagnosis.

Slide 5-52   **Scenario 6—Field Diagnosis and Treatment Options**
- ▶ Discuss the treatment options. Acknowledge variances for local protocols.
- ▶ Brochodilators are appropriate. Continue to monitor cardiac status. For CHF, the initial concern is to decrease preload and afterload. Nitroglycerin is the best choice.
- ▶ This patient would be a candidate for CPAP or BiPAP.

Slide 5-53   **Summary**
- ▶ Summarize: Focus on the importance of dyspnea as a life-threat and treating aggressively.

⊞ CHAPTER 6: CHEST DISCOMFORT OR PAIN

SLIDE NO.   **SLIDE TITLE/NOTES**

Slide 6-1   **Chest Discomfort**
- ▶ Acute coronary syndrome (ACS) may have many presentations (tightness, etc.), not just pain.
- ▶ Patients with ACS may deny "pain" but complain of ache, pressure, tightness, or heaviness.
- ▶ Chest pain or discomfort should immediately invoke thoughts of ACS or acute myocardial infarction (AMI).
- ▶ However, there are many other causes of chest pain, which will be reviewed as part of this presentation.

Slide 6-2   **Introduction**
- ▶ Up to 5% of all patients who turn out to have AMI are initially discharged from the ED even after EKG, chest radiograph, and lab evaluations.
- ▶ Because of this, every chest pain is initially treated as a serious condition.

Slide 6-3   **Anatomy and Physiology**
- ▶ Emphasize that chest pain can originate outside of the chest.

Slide 6-4   **Thoracic Structures**
- ▶ Review the structures of the chest.
- ▶ Any disease process that affects structures lying within the thoracic cavity can produce chest pain.

Slide 6-5   **Types of Chest Pain**
- ▶ Somatic: Pain that originates from nerve fibers located in the skin or parietal pleura.
- ▶ Visceral: Pain that originates from pain fibers in organs or the visceral pleura.

Slide 6-6   **Assessment Priorities**
- ▶ History and physical exam will be key to identifying the cause of chest pain.

Slide 6-7   **Focused History**
- ▶ Review the SAMPLE. Encourage participants to focus on the type of chest pain and history of risk factors for various conditions.

Slide 6-8   **Causes of Chest Pain**
- ▶ Address the causes of chest pain, life-threatening vs. non-life-threatening.
- ▶ Do not discuss each in detail.

Slide 6-9   **Management Priorities**
- ▶ Emphasize timely treatment and prompt transport.

Slide 6-10   **General Management Priorities for Patients with Chest Pain**
- ▶ Review

Slide 6-11   **Scenario 1—Scene Size-up**
- ▶ Allow participants to call out their responses.
- ▶ Reinforce: Location, patient positioning, onset, age of patient, and types of problems to anticipate.

SLIDE NO.	SLIDE TITLE/NOTES	NOTES

▶ The scene is safe.

▶ Summarize by reporting that the initial assessment indicates a potentially critical patient.

Slide 6-12   Scenario 1—Initial Assessment

▶ Discuss any factors not brought out in the previous slide.

▶ Reinforce chronic vs. acute, potential for multiple problems, and the need for additional assessment, which transitions to the next slide.

▶ Discuss initial management to include oxygen and IV, cardiac monitor and 12 lead EKG.

Slide 6-13   Scenario 1—Focused History

▶ Discuss the findings and potential differential/field diagnoses.

Slide 6-14   Scenario 1—Focused History

▶ Discuss the findings.

Slide 6-15   Scenario 1—Focused Physical Exam

▶ Discuss the findings and generate differential field diagnoses. If asked, BP 80/60 on the left, but difficult to hear.

Slide 6-16   Scenario 1—Discussion

▶ Discuss the potential differential field diagnoses and the process (pertinent negatives, rule outs, physical findings, onset) they used to come to the diagnosis.

Slide 6-17   Scenario 1—Field Diagnosis and Treatment Options

▶ Discuss the treatment options. Acknowledge variances for local protocols.

Slide 6-18   Aortic Dissection Discussion

▶ Discuss the common findings and risk factors associated with aortic dissection.

Slide 6-19   Scenario 2—Scene Size-up

▶ Allow participants to call out their responses.

▶ Reinforce: Location, patient positioning, onset, age of patient, and types of problems to anticipate.

▶ The scene is safe.

▶ Summarize by reporting that the initial assessment indicates a potentially critical patient.

Slide 6-20   Scenario 2—Initial Assessment

▶ Discuss any factors not brought out in the previous slide.

▶ Reinforce chronic vs. acute, potential for multiple problems, and the need for additional assessment, which transitions to the next slide.

▶ Discuss initial management to include oxygen and IV, cardiac monitor and 12 lead EKG.

Slide 6-21   Scenario 2—Focused History

▶ Discuss the findings and potential differential/field diagnoses.

Slide 6-22   Scenario 2—Focused History

▶ Discuss the findings.

Slide 6-23   Scenario 2—Focused Physical Exam

▶ Discuss the findings and generate differential field diagnoses.

SLIDE NO.	SLIDE TITLE/NOTES
Slide 6-24	**Scenario 2—Discussion** ▶ Discuss the potential differential Field Diagnoses and the process (pertinent negatives, rule outs, physical findings, onset) they used to come to the diagnosis.
Slide 6-25	**Scenario 2—Field Diagnosis and Treatment Options** ▶ Discuss the treatment options. Acknowledge variances for local protocols.
Slide 6-26	**Esophageal Rupture** ▶ Discuss the common findings and risk factors associated with esophageal rupture.
Slide 6-27	**Scenario 3—Scene Size-up** ▶ Allow participants to call out their responses. ▶ Reinforce: Location, patient positioning, onset, age of patient and types of problems to anticipate. ▶ The scene is safe. ▶ Summarize by reporting that the initial assessment indicates a potentially critical patient.
Slide 6-28	**Scenario 3—Initial Assessment** ▶ Discuss any factors not brought out in the previous slide. ▶ Reinforce chronic vs. acute, potential for multiple problems, and the need for additional assessment, which transitions to the next slide. ▶ Discuss initial management to include oxygen and IV, cardiac monitor and 12 lead EKG.
Slide 6-29	**Scenario 3—Focused History** ▶ Discuss the findings and potential differential/field diagnoses.
Slide 6-30	**Scenario 3—Focused History** ▶ Discuss the findings.
Slide 6-31	**Scenario 3—Focused Physical Exam** ▶ Discuss the findings and generate differential field diagnoses.
Slide 6-32	**Scenario 3—Discussion** ▶ Discuss the potential differential field diagnoses and the process (pertinent negatives, rule outs, physical findings, and onset) they used to come to the diagnosis.
Slide 6-33	**Scenario 3—Field Diagnosis and Treatment Options** ▶ Discuss the treatment options. Acknowledge variances for local protocols.
Slide 6-34	**Pericarditis** ▶ Discuss the common findings and risk factors associated with pericarditis.
Slide 6-35	**Pericarditis** ▶ Describe the common 12 lead ECG changes for pericarditis.
Slide 6-36	**Scenario 4—Scene Size-up** ▶ Allow participants to call out their responses.

SLIDE NO.	SLIDE TITLE/NOTES	NOTES

▶ Reinforce: Location, patient positioning, onset, age of patient, and types of problems to anticipate.

▶ The scene is safe.

▶ Summarize by reporting that the initial assessment indicates a potentially critical patient.

Slide 6-37   **Scenario 4—Initial Assessment**

▶ Discuss any factors not brought out in the previous slide.

▶ Reinforce chronic vs. acute, potential for multiple problems, and the need for additional assessment, which transitions to the next slide.

▶ Discuss initial management to include oxygen and IV, cardiac monitor and 12 lead EKG.

Slide 6-38   **Scenario 3—Focused History**

▶ Discuss the findings and potential differential/field diagnoses.

Slide 6-39   **Scenario 4—Focused History**

▶ Discuss the findings.

Slide 6-40   **Scenario 4—Focused Physical Exam**

▶ Discuss the findings and generate differential field diagnoses.

Slide 6-41   **Scenario 4—Discussion**

▶ Discuss the potential differential field diagnoses and the process (pertinent negatives, rule outs, physical findings, onset) they used to come to the diagnosis.

Slide 6-42   **Scenario 4—Field Diagnosis and Treatment Options**

▶ Discuss the treatment options. Acknowledge variances for local protocols.

▶ NSTEMI (Non-ST Elevation MI [ST depression in V1 and 2])

▶ ACS (may represent an acute posterior wall myocardial infarction)

Slide 6-43   **Acute Coronary Syndrome**

▶ Discuss the common findings and risk factors associated with acute coronary syndrome (AMI–STEMI and NSTEMI).

Slide 6-44   **Summary**

▶ Ask for questions and summarize.

▦ CHAPTER 7: ALTERED MENTAL STATUS (SEIZURE, HEADACHES, AND SYNCOPE)

SLIDE	SLIDE TITLE/NOTES

Slide 7-1   **Introduction**
- ▸ Introduce altered mental status lecture.
- ▸ Stress the importance of an organized approach to all cases of altered mental status because signs and symptoms can often be very subtle.

Slide 7-2   **AMS Defined**
- ▸ Altered mental status is any deviation from "normal" level of consciousness.
- ▸ It is a significant finding for a more severe underlying condition.
- ▸ Emphasize the need for the caregiver to use his or her experience and instincts for possible causes of AMS.
- ▸ It is not a disease, but can be an ominous sign of an underlying life threat. The assessment and management focus is to develop an initial impression and move to "rule in/rule out" possibilities. While gathering historical information, narrow the focus to probabilities to determine a differential field diagnosis.
- ▸ Focus on the difference between the life threats and non-life threats.

Slide 7-3   **AMS Anatomy**
- ▸ The brain is the primary source for altered mental status.
- ▸ Forces outside the brain can also cause AMS.
- ▸ Emphasize intracranial and extracranial causes of AMS.
- ▸ Discuss structural causes, metabolic causes, and toxic causes.

Slide 7-4   **The Cerebrum (diagram)**
- ▸ Discuss the different lobes of the brain, and their basic functions.
- ▸ The majority of AMS and comatose states are explained with reference to dysfunction of the RAS and/or the cerebrum.
- ▸ Cerebrum maintains a state of awakeness; the RAS maintains states of arousal/awakeness; that is, the lights are on but no one is home.
- ▸ The cerebrum is the "awareness"—the lights are on; the RAS is the "awakeness"—no one is home.
- ▸ A person with an intact RAS and two cerebral hemispheres has full orientation.
- ▸ Dysfunction of both cerebral hemispheres means serious alteration in mentation.
- ▸ If one hemisphere is dysfunctional, the patient is conscious/aware but has behavioral changes and/or loss of neurological ability.
- ▸ Example: CVA where damage in one hemisphere exhibits confusion and impaired motor/sensory on the opposite side of infarct.

Slide 7-5   **Scenario I**

- ▶ Discuss the importance of ruling in/out trauma as you approach.
- ▶ Recognize the need to conduct organized initial and detailed physical examinations in all cases of AMS.
- ▶ What are the possible causes of seizures? Ask the participants to outline possible causes of seizures, and management for BLS and ALS alike.
- ▶ Seizures and seizure disorders are among the oldest recorded diseases.
- ▶ It is a recurrent disorder of cerebral function with a rapid onset that is characterized by brief attacks of consciousness alteration, motor activity, sensory phenomena, or inappropriate behavior caused by abnormal discharge of cerebral neurons.
- ▶ To this day, seizures are poorly understood by the medical community.
- ▶ There is a relatively new classification system to the terminology of seizures. The two main classes of seizures are generalized seizures and partial seizures. Each of these is subdivided into additional classes and is based on whether the patient loses consciousness or not.
  - — Generalized seizures used to be called grand mal, petit mal, minor motor, etc. They are bilaterally symmetrical, involving both hemispheres, and include uncontrolled neural activity with loss of consciousness. The subcategories may include the absence seizure (pediatric) and tonic-clonic seizure.
  - — Tonic-clonic: Dramatic, rapid loss of consciousness that may be accompanied by a loud cry. Tonic spasms will last 10–30 seconds, then clonic (contraction and relaxation) activity will begin symmetrically and can last up to 30 minutes.
- ▶ A postical phase can last for minutes to hours and mimic stroke in the early phase.
- ▶ Partial seizures used to be called focal motor seizures, Jacksonian seizures, temporal lobe seizures, and psychomotor seizures. They involve neurons from only one hemisphere and do not include loss of consciousness.
  - — Simple partial seizures can include motor, sensory, and autonomic signs but no change in consciousness. There is little or no postical phase. Patients with simple partial seizures are able to interpret and answer questions and follow commands.
  - — Complex partial and episodic changes in behavior—looks like a psychiatric emergency. Usually begins with an aura and includes minor muscle tremors. These patients are unable to follow commands and have little ability to focus.

Slide 7-6   **Possibilities and Differentials**

- ▶ It is important for the participants to look at each cause broadly on possibilities and then to narrow focus through differentials. Altered mental status has many possible causes.

▶ Consider structural, intracranial, and extracranial. What could this scenario be due to? It is a seizure due to hypoglycemia. Continue to query the participants on this.

▶ Have the participants try to narrow down the cause based on the information provided.

Slide 7-7   **Scenario I Initial Assessment**

▶ Conduct the initial assessments in a systematic manner.

▶ Look for clues as you approach, and question family, bystanders, and other EMS responders.

▶ What is your first impression as you approach the scene? Stable or unstable?

▶ Consider the different causes of AMS, and ask the participants what may be the cause in this case.

Slide 7-8   **Scenario I Cont.**

▶ Now that the students have more information on the vital signs, try to determine the cause.

▶ Do the vital signs indicate a more precise diagnosis? Not yet; however, the information obtained in the next slide should have the participants looking more closely at the blood glucose level.

▶ What is the cause of the low GCS score, and how should it be managed? It is important to consider a more definitive airway; however, an advanced airway without correcting the blood glucose would be improper.

▶ Ensure that BLS and ALS providers recognize the need for early airway control, and supplemental O_2 delivery.

Slide 7-9   **Scenario I Focused History and Focused Medial Assessment**

▶ Unable to obtain due to LOC and no bystander assistance.

▶ Ask the participants what the cause of the patchy ecchymosis indicates. See if they are aware of the possibility of diabetes.

▶ Discuss the possibilities of trauma, liver dysfunction, and bleeding disorders as differentials.

▶ Ask if the history indicates a seizure disorder, or if the seizure has another etiology.

▶ Point out the improvement of O_2 saturation, and the decrease in $EtCO_2$.

Slide 7-10   **Scenario I Management**

▶ IV site initiated. What is your plan for fluid resuscitation?

▶ Stress the importance of a second secure IV site, because a constant medication route is critical in cases of AMS. A second site is a secure back-up in the event one is lost due to handling, patient movement, etc. Also, some medications, fluids, and blood products given prehospital may require separate lines.

▶ Indicate the need for blood sampling for blood glucose level measurements.

▶ Also important is the appropriate gauge catheter and vein for the delivery of D50.

▶ Discuss the possible use of glucagon for advanced EMT providers, and its "back-up" possibilities in the unlikely event of IV failure.

▶ Talk about oral glucose administration and airway patency.

Slide 7-11 **Blood Glucose**

▶ Blood glucose measurement is relatively simple to measure, and should be done in all cases of altered mental status.

▶ Recognize the need to repeat blood glucose measurements when the patient is found in compensatory shock. Blood glucose readings can be artificially high in these cases, and should be repeated in longer transport situations.

▶ Ask the patient or family member to provide you with the patient's own glucometer. What does the history in their device indicate? Is it calibrated and similar to the measurements in your device? Reviewing the patient's glucometer can show you trends and the frequency of their tests. It is a fair indicator of how responsible the patient is to his/her diabetes. Calibration of EMS glucometers to read venous blood is important, because many samples are acquired from IV sharps, a common, but not recommended practice. Medical personnel should understand the formula to covert blood glucose levels from mg/dl to mmol/l (mg/dl ÷ 18 = mmol/L or mmol/L × 18 = mg/d).

▶ Ensure that the participants understand that not all glucometers are compatible with venous blood samples from IV sharps.

▶ Although commonly done, sampling from a sharp is not without its risks in the moving ambulance. BSI must be considered at all times.

Slide 7-12 **Diabetic Patients**

▶ Discuss the four main types of diabetic emergencies: hypoglycemia, DKA, hyperglycemia, and hyperosmolar hyperglycemic non-ketotic syndrome (HHNS).

▶ Discuss the similarities of these crises, and the preponderance of hypoglycemia due to its rapid onset, often missed by the patients themselves.

▶ Discuss how infection and illness can predispose the diabetic patient to DKA or hyperglycemia, even in the well-managed diabetic patient.

▶ Discuss the 3 p's of diabetes: polyuria, polyphagia, and polydipsia.

▶ Also discuss how almost 50% of diabetics are undiagnosed type II, and that this problem is growing in developed countries like the United States and Canada.

Slide 7-13 **Diabetic Patients Cont.**

▶ Talk to participants about the rates of onset for the four types of diabetes discussed.

▶ Many patients are unaware of their diabetic history, and how history-taking is important in diagnosing this.

▶ Talk about the importance of detailed physical examinations, and how clues in assessment can lead you to a diabetic patient. Encourage participants to look for the bruising, toughening, or scarring of repeated injection sites, and signs of microcirculatory failure such as diabetic foot changes.

▶ Male diabetics are more likely to require amputations due to diabetes than female patients.

▶ Discuss scarring, bruising, and tissue changed from long-term injections of exogenous insulin.

Slide 7-14   **Scenario I Summary**

▶ The recognition of a hypoglycemic state indicates the patient's seizure is most likely due to hypoglycemia.

▶ Ensure that participants consider that the genesis of the seizure may be unrelated to the hypoglycemia as well, and that thorough assessments, diagnostics, and history-taking can reduce the likelihood of missing critical components.

▶ Discuss the importance of on-going assessment, frequent reassessments as needed, and delivery to an appropriate facility.

▶ After arrival at the local hospital, and meeting with the patient's parents, it was discovered that he has experienced seizures before due to drops in his blood glucose, and improper management of diet.

▶ Differential Diagnosis: Generalized seizure related to hypoglycemia.

Slide 7-15   **Scenario II**

▶ Scene safety and looking for clues are important in this case.

▶ Airway maintenance is paramount in this patient, and critical to manage respirations and the pathological respiratory pattern.

▶ Investigate clues surrounding the patient's recent medical history, and query the family in detail if time allows.

▶ Apply appropriate BSI and consider the possibility of an infectious agent.

Slide 7-16   **Possibilities and Differentials**

▶ It is important that the participants look at each cause broadly and then focus through the differentials. Altered mental status has many possible causes.

▶ Consider structural, intracranial, and extracranial. What could this scenario be due to? This patient is suffering from an intracranial infection. Continue to query the participants, but do not provide the answer yet.

▶ Have the participants try to narrow down the cause based on the information provided.

Slide 7-17   **Scenario II Initial Assessment**

▶ Really emphasize the need to query the scene and the family members in this case.

▶ It is critical to deal with the airway compromise as soon as possible, and to manage the pathological respiratory pattern with positive pressure ventilation and tracheal intubation or other airway techniques.

▶ Ask the participants why the patient is pale and dry. This patient is febrile and dehydrated, with no additional moisture to produce diaphoresis. Discussion can ensue on the importance of providing fluids, and the allowance of passive cooling in the absence of diaphoresis.

Slide 7-18 **Scenario II Cont.**

▶ What does the presence of the Cheyne-Stokes respiratory pattern indicate? This pathological respiratory pattern is evidence of the severity of the patient's condition.

▶ Discuss the significance of pathological respiratory patterns, and the need to support the ABCs in these cases.

▶ Why is the pulse and blood pressure so high? What can we do to manage these values? The increase in blood pressure is a manifestation of cerebral perfusion compensation due to the increase in ICP. Increases in pulse rates can be traced to the increase in body temperature. Pulses increase by 20 beats per minute for every degree increase in body temperature in Fahrenheit.

▶ How do we manage the blood pressure? We leave it alone until we determine the cause. It is important to recognize that hypertension is often critical to maintain cerebral perfusion, and that pharmacological means to reduce BP may have a deleterious effect, and possibly cause further brain damage or death.

▶ Critical to refer to local protocol or medical control guidelines in these cases.

▶ Controlled transport of ventilators with continuous waveform monitoring of CO_2 and SpO_2 are recommended in these patients.

▶ Discuss the cardiac dysrhythmia, and try to determine if it is primary or secondary in this case. Should it be corrected pharmacologically or will it abate with O_2 administration? It is important to try to correct the cardiac abnormalities by allowing the O_2 administration to take effect.

Slide 7-19 **Scenario II Focused Medical Assessment**

▶ Discuss the improvements with O_2 administration and also the difficulties in this patient in regards to pathological breathing patterns.

Slide 7-20 **Scenario II Management**

▶ Tracheal intubation achieved without medications. Discuss how obtunded a patient must be in this case.

▶ Correlate the LOC with the severity of the cerebral abcess rupture.

▶ Discuss the possible meningitis/encephalitis with the rupture of the cerebral abscesses.

▶ Emphasize the need to solicit history from the family members.

▶ Differential diagnosis: Cerebral abscess related to recent nasal surgery.

Slide 7-21 **Scenario II Summary**

▶ Patients will often discontinue medications such as antibiotics early.

▶ Identify the ramifications of early discontinuation of these important medications, and the possibility of infections, or worsening infections.

▶ Nasal trauma, mastoid trauma, or surgeries can lead to infections of the brain or meninges.

► Wrap up this case with the importance of BLS and need for early ALS intervention for airway maintenance.

► Transport to appropriate hospital is critical to patient's outcome.

Slide 7-22 AMS Management

► Review of standardized approach to patient surveys, especially initial and detailed physical examinations.

► History-taking is the key to solving problems, and leading the caregiver to a possible diagnosis.

► Take this time to review the similarities from the previous two cases. This would include the importance of thorough history-taking. In situations of patient unconsciousness, the caregiver must rely on complete patient surveys, vital signs, and diagnostics.

Slide 7-23 AMS Management Cont.

► Continue discussion from previous slide, and emphasize the roles of BLS and ALS providers in areas of airway management.

► Use this opportunity to recall information from the airway management lecture and discuss medication-facilitated intubations.

► Also talk about the importance of using all diagnostic tools in patient management such as: $EtCO_2$, SpO_2, and ECG, and the importance and underutilization of body temperature.

Slide 7-24 Scenario III

► Ask the class if they work metro or rural. Consider the distance and the time from appropriate care.

► It is also noteworthy to consider the time of day, and the possible differentials such as: paroxysmal nocturnal dyspnea (PND).

► Discuss any challenges of longer dispatch times to the scene, and the severity of the patient in such remote locations.

Slide 7-25 Possibilities and Differentials

► It is important for the participant to look at each cause broadly and then to focus through differentials. Altered mental status has many possible causes.

► Consider structural, intracranial, and extracranial. What could this scenario be due to?

► Have the participants try to narrow down the cause based on the information provided. Consider the time of day and the age of the patient. It is often a respiratory call with cardiac complications that come in the early morning hours, such as PND.

Slide 7-26 Scenario III Initial Assessment

► Are there any obvious clues from the scene? The fact that the patient was too weak to make it to the bed, and collapsed with severe pulmonary edema, highlights the severity of his distress. Ask the participants for their thoughts on this.

► The initial assessment of the patient points out the severity of the condition. Ensure that delegation of all crew members take place.

▶ Irregularity of the pulse may be a primary or a secondary event. Ask the participants for their input on this significant finding.

▶ What is the cause of the shock? Is this a respiratory event, or a cardiac event with respiratory complications? This is a patient with cardiac problems, who experienced a severe and sudden onset of pulmonary edema.

▶ AMS can be caused by extracranial events not directly associated with the CNS such as the pulmonary and circulatory systems.

Slide 7-27   **Scenario III Cont.**

▶ Ensure that participants recognize the significance of early and definitive airway management.

▶ Note that this airway can initially be managed with BLS providers.

▶ The patient in this case lived in a very rural setting, and was 30 minutes from a community type hospital. Intubation and ventilations would lead to a ventilator in-hospital, and transport a further 3 hours for admission to a more suitable facility. The decision to allow the medications to work was based partly on the isolation of this case. Intubation gear was on standby; however, the patient improved remarkably with furosemide and the inhaled beta-agonists. Although both approaches could have been appropriate, it is desirable to avoid intubations if at all possible to minimize the risk of infection and dependence on the tube. Ensure that local protocols and medical control guidelines are followed in these cases.

— Recognize that this is an isolated case pertaining to the rural environment.

— Encourage discussion with the improvements of saturation and $EtCO_2$ values with supplemental O_2 and medications via nebulizer mask.

Slide 7-28   **Scenario III—Focused Medical Assessment**

▶ Encourage discussion surrounding the physical findings on this patient: the old sternotomy scar, wet lung sounds.

▶ Also consider this important point: Syncope that occurs while seated or laying down is often cardiac in origin, and is often referred to as Cardiac Syncope.

▶ The recent history indicates that the patient likely has a respiratory infection, complicated by his cardiac and respiratory problems.

▶ Discuss the need to provide furosemide to this patient.

▶ Also discuss the need to catheterize this patient prehospital if allowed by local protocols.

▶ This patient will need to void en route, and volumes will provide useful information on the effectiveness of diuretic administration.

Slide 7-29   **Scenario III Management**

▶ The IV is important for the delivery of medications.

▶ CPAP and BiPAP are also important tools in the management of these cases. Ambulance services currently carry these devices, and it is another tool to prevent intubation if possible.

▶ Discuss the possible pharmacological options with the class, especially the effects of furosemide. Diuretics are very effective in the removal of excess fluids in this case; however, it can lead to a drop in blood pressure and the need for the hospital to correct electrolytes, etc.

▶ Talk about beta-agonist medications such as Ventolin and Combivent type options. Atrovent-Ventolin (Combivent) can help with their synergistic effects, as well as Ventolin/Albuterol/Salbutamol. Combivent medications are administered only once or twice in the prehospital setting, with beta-agonists being repeated as necessary, or as per protocol.

Slide 7-30   **AMS Causes Review**

▶ It is a good time to reflect on the causes of AMS with the class.

▶ Emphasize that AMS has many causes, direct and indirect, in reference to the CNS.

Slide 7-31   **AMS Causes Defined**

▶ Discuss the different types of stroke.

▶ Occlusive strokes cause blockage in arteries. This insult usually affects motor, sensory, and speech areas versus significant mental status changes.

▶ The signs and symptoms worsen progressively, but can often stabilize in 24–72 hours (in 80–85% of cases).

▶ Often present with nausea, vomiting, hemiplegia, hemiparesis, aphasia, and dysphasia.

▶ Thrombotic—is a clot in an artery. This occlusion develops gradually because ischemia is present long before total blockage. Generally occurs at rest.

▶ Anti-coagulants and antiplatelets can prevent thrombosis formation. Often a history of angina.

▶ Pupils may be dilated on the affected side and tend to gaze away from the affected side. This is usually due to tumor/bleeding with mass effect.

▶ Embolic incidents generally occur in the carotid artery. This is why checking for bruits prior to carotid massage can help to avoid strokes. These incidents are often due to atrial fibrillation.

▶ Generally numbness opposite the lesion.

▶ Vertigo, diplopia, and hemiparesis are common symptoms.

▶ Talk about the trend to discuss strokes as "brain attacks" to encourage a more prompt public and EMS response.

▶ It is very important to talk about fibrinolytic therapy in the management of the stroke patient.

▶ Zero hour begins from the onset of stroke symptoms (last time patient known to be normal). The 3-hour window is the current recommendation because after 3 hours reperfusion of cerebral tissue can cause deleterious effects.

▶ Hemorraghic stroke history typically involves a history of hypertension, smoking, and recent exertion.

▶ Differential diagnosis: Cardiopulmonary complication which causes alteration in mentation.

Slide 7-32 CVA—Stroke—Brain Attack

Slide 7-33 **CVA Management Considerations**
- ▶ Solicit feedback from the class on their local guidelines for the management of stroke patients.
- ▶ Apply current stroke assessment test.
- ▶ Ask if fibrinolytic therapy is being used in their regions.
- ▶ Discuss the importance of blood glucose measurements, and how dextrose may be replaced if absolutely necessary.
- ▶ Also noteworthy is CVA-induced hypertension as a compensatory mechanism to maintain cerebral perfusion. Discuss how previous management included pharmacological treatment to lower BP, and what potential damage that may cause, by actually producing cerebral ischemia due to decreased blood flow to the affected neural tissue.

Slide 7-34 **Meningitis and Encephalitis**
- ▶ Assess the condition and treat life threats as per usual.
- ▶ Determine if dehydration exists and treat accordingly, but cautiously as well.
- ▶ Observe for fluid overload.
- ▶ Consider the use of transport ventilators and $EtCO_2$ monitoring.

Slide 7-35 **pH and Altered Mental Status**
- ▶ Talk about the importance of pH in normal cellular activity.
- ▶ Discuss the normal pH range of 7.35–7.45.
- ▶ Also talk about the trend of ALS providers using blood gas analysis equipment in the prehospital care arena.
- ▶ Paramedics and nurses should be aware of pH values and blood gas analysis, and the techniques and equipment to do so.
- ▶ Compare and contrast respiratory and metabolic acidosis causes.

Slide 7-36 **pH and Altered Mental Status**
- ▶ Assessment of these disturbances include:
  - — Scene size-up evaluation for history of use of cigarettes, multiple medications, drug paraphernalia, evidence of diabetes or renal failure, poor living conditions, malnutrition.
  - — Facial affect in acidosis is often lethargy; in alkalosis, hyperactivity.
  - — Assessment of ABCs includes evaluation of respiratory patterns and administration of oxygen and/or ventilation.
  - — Chief complaint of lethargy, weakness, confusion, kidney dialysis, COPD, and chest pain in acidosis.
  - — Chief complaints of muscular spasticity, ataxia, numbness and tingling in extremities, dizziness, diarrhea or vomiting prior to illness, and inappropriate behavior in alkalosis.
  - — SAMPLE history includes usage of other medications, last oral intake, and history of vomiting. Assess for gradual or sudden onset to determine severity.
  - — Physical exam includes evaluation of mucosa for hydration, carpal pedal spasm (alkalosis), and delay in capillary refill (alkalosis). Vital signs may vary.

    — In acidosis, pulses remain normal or slightly elevated and as symptoms worsen become weaker and slower.

    — Alkalosis typically presents with elevated pulses.

▶ Definitive treatment may not be accomplished in the field and may be directed at management of life threats only.

▶ For respiratory acidosis and alkalosis, oxygen and ventilation are appropriate.

▶ Respiratory acidosis may include bronchodilators for COPD and naloxone for overdose. If fluid accumulates in lungs from pneumonia or infectious disease, the patient can be placed in High Fowlers to allow gravity to help drain fluid and improve gas exchange.

▶ BVM can be used to assist excretion of CO_2.

▶ In respiratory alkalosis, coach the patient to decrease respirations to help decrease pH by closing mouth and breathing through nose.

▶ Treat cardiac dysrhythmias per AHA recommendations. In metabolic acidosis administration of sodium bicarbonate IVP, 1 mEq/kg may be appropriate.

▶ IV therapy should remain TKO in an effort not to dilute electrolyte concentrations. Arterial blood gases (ABGs) should be obtained for more definitive diagnosis and management.

▶ Two of the major contributors to acid-base imbalance are disturbances in sodium and calcium.

▶ Sodium—primary cation in extracellular fluid. Distributes water and also is responsible for waste removal and thermoregulation.

▶ Normal values are 135–145 mEq/l. Hypernatremia increases intravascular osmolarity, causing cellular dehydration.

▶ The shrinkage of cells affects the size of the brain cells and can actually decrease the size of the brain itself. This condition alters nerve depolarization, causing irritability and seizures.

▶ Hyponatremia causes extracellular shifts into intracellular spaces, causing edema.

▶ The edema results in increased ICP and decreased cerebral perfusion.

▶ Typical symptoms include headache, stupor and seizure, pathologic respiratory patterns, facial palsy/droop, tongue deviation, aphasia, vision and pupil changes, and NVD.

▶ May be taking potassium supplements, diuretics, digitalis, beta blockers, and thiazides.

▶ Calcium—A cation stored in bones and teeth that maintains cell membrane stability. This cation regulates calcium entry in cell, blood clotting mechanisms, nerve and muscle impulses, and myocardial contraction.

▶ Normal ranges are 9–10 mg/dl.

▶ Hypercalcemia—Increases permeability to sodium and decreases electrical impulse conduction, diminishing CNS function.

▶ Decreased neurotransmission causes seizures, muscle weakness, decreased myocardial automaticity leading to severe heart blocks, decreased cardiac output, and decreased cerebral perfusion.

▶ Symptoms include hyperactive parathyroid (which regulates calcium), shortened QT and ST segments, shallow respirations, chest pain, and syncopal episodes.

▶ Hypocalcaemia allows sodium to enter cell and increase depolarization.

▶ Patients exhibit tetany, convulsions, prolonged QT and ST segments, decreased myocardial contractions, pulmonary congestion, and poor peripheral perfusion.

▶ Field management focuses on managing life threats and rapid transport for definitive diagnosis and treatment.

▶ Review the primary causes such as: respiratory acidosis being caused by impaired pulmonary ventilation, metabolic acidosis from increases in metabolic acid production, or decreases in bicarbonate.

Slide 7-37　　**pH & AMS**

▶ Respiratory alkalosis results when CO_2 is excreted faster than it is produced.

▶ What are the possible causes, and discuss these with the class. Ask for examples that the students may have dealt with in the past.

▶ Metabolic alkalosis: discuss excess in circulating bicarbonate, and its impact on the tissues and overall pH.

Slide 7-38　　**Scenario IV**

▶ What are the hazards of this environment? Could this be a possible crime scene?

▶ This patient seems to be a "shut-in" patient, and may be suffering the effects expected in this group, such malnutrition, loneliness, and emotional issues.

▶ This patient is suffering from chronic hypothermia, induced by lifestyle and medical conditions and medications.

▶ Put this case out for discussion to solicit possible differentials from the class.

Slide 7-39　　**Possibilities and Differentials**

▶ It is important for the students to look at each cause broadly and then focus through differentials. Altered mental status has many possible causes.

▶ Consider structural, intracranial, and extracranial. What could this scenario be due to?

▶ Have the students try to narrow down the cause based on the information provided.

Slide 7-40　　**Scenario IV Initial Assessment**

▶ Talk about the extra resources on scene, and how this can work to the advantage of you and the patient.

▶ Stress the importance of thorough scene assessments in these cases where history is slight, and unavailable to communicating with the patient.

▶ Discuss airway management and the poor circulatory status. Warmed O_2 if available may be beneficial in cases of hypothermia. These devices are not common, however, in most EMS systems. Warm IV fluids are also desirable, but difficult as the fluids cool as they travel through the tubing.

▶ Focus on the possible diagnosis, and try to rule out previous differentials listed by the class.

Slide 7-41   **Scenario IV Cont.**

▶ Do these vital signs focus your assessment? It should point the participant to a diagnosis of decreased metabolic activity, and possible chronic hypothermia.

▶ What are the factors producing such diminished vital signs? Hypothermia caused by decreased metabolic state.

▶ Could these vital signs point to overdose, underdose, or cardiac problems leading to mental status changes?

▶ Encourage discussion of this patient's condition and solicit feedback on the elderly living alone in the participant's service area.

▶ What can EMS providers do as a patient advocate in such situations? EMS could get involved in calling local "high-risk" elders, checking in by phone or in person.

Slide 7-42   **Scenario IV Focused Medical Assessment**

▶ The goiter likely indicates a thyroid abnormality. Ask the participant if this changes anything in their assessments. What medications do thyroid patients take, and what are the side effects? Thyroxin can produce arrythmias, cramps, diarrhea, nervousness, tachycardia, and tremors. Propranolol is considered in cases of thyroxin overdoses. Estrogen can also decrease the bioavailabilty of thyroxin by increasing binding proteins.

▶ Could metabolic imbalance be causing these vital signs?

▶ Do you take body temperatures in your service? It is important as a vital sign, and especially in this case of chronic hypothermia.

▶ What is the significance of the outdated thyroxin? There is always the risk of the drug not working at all, or possibly causing toxic effects.

Slide 7-43   **Scenario IV Management**

▶ Now that IV access and intubation has been achieved, is pharmacology an option? Not likely in this case due to the hypothermic condition. Drugs are not properly taken up by the tissues, and often remain in the circulatory system during hypothermic states. Once the patient is rewarmed, these drugs become metabolically active and can produce overdose situations.

▶ *Differential Diagnosis:* Abnormal thyroid function related to hypothermia and poor nutrition (failure to thrive).

▶ This patient is hypothermic, and movements must be done gently. Moving the hypothermic patient can result in serious cardiac dysrhythmias.

▶ Chronic hypothermia can occur in almost every region in the world, and this is relatively common.

Slide 7-44   **Scenario IV Cont.**

▶ Use this opportunity to review hypothermia, and the vulnerability of seniors to these conditions due to decreased metabolic rates; pre-existing medical conditions; the use of medications; poor nutrition; and the general inability to thrive due to fixed and low incomes.

▶ Heating costs, food, and the desire to live independently can produce these problems in a large part of our population.

▶ EMS can take a pro-active preventative approach to high-risk patients living in their service areas, and could take the lead on this initiative.

Slide 7-45   Scenario IV Summary

▶ Talk about cardiac dysrhythmias produced in hypothermia such as VF and VT.

▶ Talk and discuss current ECC-AHA guidelines for management of hypothermia and cardiac arrest.

▶ Talk about the risk of overdose of IV-administered medications as patient becomes more "metabolically active."

Slide 7-46   Thyroid Disorders

▶ The thyroid gland is part of the endocrine (ductless) system.

▶ The hormones it produces and secretes are related to the patient's metabolic rates.

▶ Overproduction and underproduction of thyroid hormones can lead to AMS problems.

▶ Millions of North Americans, and people worldwide, are on thyroid replacement therapy, and need to have their levels checked on a regular basis.

▶ Consider that half of the thyroid can be removed and that the remaining half may or may not maintain adequate production and release of thyroid hormones.

Slide 7-47   Thyroid Disorders Cont.

▶ Hypothyroidism is the most common thyroid disorder.

▶ These patients may be overweight, intolerant of the cold, and may also present as edematous, moon face.

▶ These patients require levothyroxine or Synthroid to supplement or replace the function of their thyroid gland.

▶ The most severe cases may result in bradycardias, CHF produced from these poor heart rates, and lower cardiac output.

▶ Palpate the neck for the presence of a goiter, or surgical scar indicating thyroidectomy.

Slide 7-48   Thyroid Disorders Cont.

▶ Hyperthyroidism increases metabolic activity. It may be produced by a benign or malignant growth affecting the thyroid gland itself.

▶ Look for increases in basal metabolic rates such as tachycardias, nervousness, tremors, and anxiety.

▶ Mood changes and decreases in attention span are not uncommon signs.

▶ Exopthalmos is possible as the pads behind the orbits become edematous, producing this "bulging" of the eyes.

▶ Consider that the patient may be taking too much exogenous levothyroxine.

▶ When did the patient last see his/her physician, and have the TSH levels evaluated? This can be a teachable moment for EMS providers.

▶ Monitor blood glucose levels, because hypoglycemia may result from excessive use of ATP energy and glucose. Often these patients are prescribed propylthiovracil and methimazole (Tapazole).

Slide 7-49

Thyroid Disorders Cont.

▶ Myxedema coma is a very severe hypothyroid complication.

▶ CNS depression causes include: cold, stress, infection, and the use of CNS depressants.

▶ This is a severe condition with poor patient outcomes.

▶ Severe depression of other body systems can result.

Slide 7-50

Thiamine Deficiency

▶ These patients may require the administration of thiamine.

▶ Look for the Triad of Encephalopathy: disorientation, gait ataxia, and occulomotor dysfunction.

▶ Thiamine is essential in the conversion of dextrose into ATP within the cells.

▶ Providing dextrose to a thiamine-deficient patient will not have the desired effect, and the patient may well remain unconscious or obtunded.

▶ 50 mg deep IM and an additional 50 or 100 mg IV may allow the dextrose to be properly converted at a cellular level.

▶ Long-term damage from thiamine deficiency can result in Korsakoff's Amnestic Syndrome. This is a permanent condition.

Slide 7-51

Management Issues

▶ As in all cases of AMS, complete surveys and diagnostics.

▶ Once blood is sampled for blood glucose level, replace dextrose with concurrent administration of thiamine.

▶ It is advised to administer thiamine 100 mg IV push.

▶ Recognize that Korsakoff's psychosis is permanent, and will not respond or change due to D50 administration.

Slide 7-52

Scenario V

▶ What is the correlation between heavy physical exertion and the initial information available in this dispatch? It is likely that this patient is suffering from a heat-related emergency, combined with excessive physical activity.

▶ What are the possible causes of this call? Consider increased metabolic activity and the conditions it may produce.

▶ This is a young patient, and that by its nature may rule out certain conditions.

Slide 7-53

Possibilities and Differentials

▶ It is important for the participants to look at each cause broadly and then focus through the differentials. Altered mental status has many possible causes.

▶ Consider structural, intracranial, and extracranial. What could this scenario be due to?

Slide 7-54 **Scenario V Initial Assessment**
- ▶ You have determined that the scene is safe and secure.
- ▶ You find this patient conscious and alert with active vomiting.
- ▶ Ensure that trauma is not a cause in this case of high-risk events. Some medical patients experience traumatic injuries as well.
- ▶ Ask the participants to list the possible causes of the shock.

Slide 7-55 **Scenario V Focused Medical Assessment.**
- ▶ Consider the challenges of O_2 administration in actively vomiting patients.
- ▶ This patient may have previously undiagnosed medical conditions.
- ▶ Encourage discussion on this possibility. Query the by-standers and other participants as to the activities being done by the patient.

Slide 7-56 **Scenario V Cont.**
- ▶ *Differential Diagnosis:* Heat exhaustion related to dehydration and electrolyte imbalance.
- ▶ Elicit discussion on these assessment pearls. Look at the skin color, condition, and temperature. Recognize that it need not be excessively warm outdoors to produce environmental conditions such as heat exhaustion.
- ▶ The importance of the headache may indicate a previous condition, or may lead the class to the diagnosis of heat exhaustion/stroke. Discuss the effects of severe perspiration without proper replacement.
- ▶ Query the class about the nutrition of this particular patient. Is the patient's diet appropriate to the exercise being done?
- ▶ Also stress the need to re-evaluate the blood glucose level when and if the vitals return to normal.
- ▶ Discuss the body temperature. What does the class think of it being slightly below normal? Discuss the fact that the patient is cooling adequately.

Slide 7-57 **Scenario V Management**
- ▶ What are your goals for IV therapy? Fluid replacement is important in these cases of heat exhaustion.
- ▶ O_2 can be supplemented via nasal cannula to actively vomiting patients.
- ▶ The patient's lack of urination indicates the severity of his dehydration.
- ▶ Do not provide anti-emetics in the absence of fluid therapy.

Slide 7-58 **Scenario V Summary**
- ▶ This patient was suffering from heat exhaustion and dehydration. Poor diet and fluid intake, as well as the heavy physical exercise, worsened the condition.
- ▶ Fluid therapy and O_2 therapy increased patient's circulatory status and began the homeostatic return.
- ▶ Heat exhaustion untreated can lead to heat stroke. Heat stroke can cause death and/or severe brain damage.

SLIDE NO.	SLIDE TITLE/NOTES

Slide 7-59 **Electrolyte Abnormalities**
- ▶ Review the four situations as listed on the slide.
- ▶ Discuss EMS limitations because values cannot be evaluated properly in the prehospital setting.

Slide 7-60 **Altered Mental Status Summary**
- ▶ Review the importance of thorough physical examinations and use all diagnostics possible.
- ▶ Continue to hone your skills in the art of history-taking, and become a detective in patient care. Ask many questions, and listen to the answers and your instincts.

CHAPTER 8: ACUTE ABDOMINAL PAIN

SLIDE NO.   **SLIDE TITLE/NOTES**

Slide 8-1   **Acute Abdominal Pain**
- ▶ Focus on the overview of the lecture. Limited epidemiology is offered for interest in the notes below.
  - — The acute abdomen accounts for 5% of ER visits and makes up approximately 1/3 of the surgical problems seen.
  - — Of the patients who present with acute abdominal pain, 15–30% will require surgery. This percentage is even higher in the elderly.
  - — This lecture will focus on identifying the sick vs. not sick, the affected system, and the potential life threats.

Slide 8-2   **Acute Abdomen**
Briefly summarize the process.

Slide 8-3   **Experiences and Knowledge**
- ▶ To come up with a differential diagnosis, you will need to connect the patient presentation to the disease process using the factors identified.
- ▶ Initially, you should identify several diagnoses and work to collect information through a thorough history and physical exam to identify a final diagnosis.
- ▶ As you work through the process, you will need to evaluate the risks and benefits of performing certain exams and treatments.
- ▶ Finally, you should constantly reassess the patient for changes and response to the treatments you have initiated.

Slide 8-4   **Keys to Abdominal Assessment**
- ▶ When assessing the abdomen, it is essential to identify life threats. You will need to look at the patient to determine if he/she is critical. Often, the assessment will require you to trust your instincts because a specific cause for the problem may not be initially apparent.
- ▶ Even though non-specific pain will account for 40–60% of the cases, it is essential that history be collected as feasible.
- ▶ Emphasize not delaying transport to obtain a diagnosis.

Slide 8-5   **Implications of Abdominal Pain**
- ▶ Knowing where the pain is located and identifying the underlying organs may assist with predicting organ involvement and identifying a diagnosis.
- ▶ If the pain is not localized, it is classified as diffuse.
- ▶ Diffuse pain or poorly localized pain felt near the midline is commonly associated with peritonitis, bowel obstruction, aortic aneurysm, gastroenteritis, and pancreatitis.

Slide 8-6   **Anatomy—Abdominal Structures**
- ▶ Allow participants to read the slide as you point out the following information:
  - — Solid organs tend to present with a constant pain.

— Hollow organs, for the most part, have the ability to contract or carry out peristalsis. Therefore, hollow organ pain is more commonly associated with crampy or colicky pain.

Slide 8-7   Anatomy—Abdominal Structures

▶ The peritoneum is the serous membrane that lines the abdominopelvic cavity. The parietal peritoneum covers the outer wall. The visceral peritoneum covers the internal organs.

▶ The peritoneum divides the abdomen vertically into the peritoneal space and the retroperitoneal space.

▶ Organs such as the kidneys, ureters, and aorta are located in the retroperitoneal space. The pancreas shares both spaces. That is why organs in the retroperitoneal space often present with back pain as opposed to anterior abdominal pain.

▶ The mesentery is a double sheet of peritoneum that supports the intestines and contains the blood vessels that supply the intestines.

▶ The skeletal structures include the vertebral column and musculature, diaphragm, and muscles of the abdominal wall.

Slide 8-8   Pain-Producing Mechanisms

▶ Distension: Pain associated with distension is usually dependent on how rapidly the distention occurs. Rapid distention causes pain, whereas slow distention usually does not cause pain.

▶ Traction: Causes pain from the tension or stretching of the tissue. It is usually caused by adhesions, distention of the common bile duct, or forceful peristalsis resulting from intestinal obstruction.

▶ Edema (or vascular congestion): Can stimulate the contraction of hollow organs causing colicky or crampy pain. The edema from inflammation can also cause painful stretching.

Slide 8-9   Pain-Producing Mechanisms

▶ Obstruction of blood vessels causes ischemic pain. Bowel obstructions stimulate pain receptors due to distention.

▶ Ischemic pain from blood vessel occlusion is steady and severe, and increases over time. Severe pain out of proportion to the findings may be from ischemia of the mesentery.

▶ Inflammation can cause pain due to the edema and/or chemicals released as part of the inflammatory response.

▶ Chemical irritation resulting from the inflammatory response releases histamine, bradykinin, and serotonin, which stimulate nerve endings causing pain.

Slide 8-10   Visceral Pain

▶ Abdominal pain has multiple origins: visceral, parietal, referred, and extra-abdominal causes. Discuss and contrast the origins of abdominal pain.

▶ Visceral pain arises from the abdominal organs and is usually located in the mid-epigastric or umbilical regions near the midline of the body.

▶ It is often diffuse, vague, and poorly localized because the nerve endings within the abdominal organs are sparse and multi-segmented. The pain is usually generated by stretch receptors. The nerve fibers enter the cord at several levels bilaterally so the patients may be unable to discriminate the exact location; thus the pain is perceived as diffuse.

▸ Solid organs produce a dull, constant pain. Hollow organs produce a crampy, colicky pain that is intermittent.

▸ Visceral pain may evolve into parietal pain as in the case of appendicitis.

Slide 8-11   **Parietal Pain**

▸ Parietal or somatic pain comes from the parietal peritoneum and is usually localized and intense.

▸ The nerve fibers from the parietal peritoneum travel with associated peripheral nerves of the spinal cord. Patients can localize the pain because the pain sensation is transmitted through specific nerve fibers on the same side and at the same dermatome level as the site of the pain. Therefore, the pain tends to be unilateral.

▸ The pain is usually sharp, discrete, constant, and localized.

▸ Patients often prefer the fetal position. If you find them supine, they will often lay with their knees drawn up. This relaxes the parietal peritoneum and helps reduce the pain. Any type of movement or activity that moves the peritoneum will increase the pain. Coughing, taking a deep breath, flexing and extending the leg, palpation, and sudden movement all may increase the pain.

▸ Parietal pain frequently occurs after visceral pain, so obtaining a history describing any change in the pain is important.

Slide 8-12   **Areas of Referred Pain**

▸ This slide and the next slide (8-13) review the anterior and posterior areas of referred pain. Review the locations.
   — Referred pain results from misinterpretation of sensory input by the brain.
   — Ovary/fallopian tube cause referred pain due to capsule's rupturing. The release of chemicals causes irritation, resulting in inflammation to the peritoneal lining, diaphragm, and phrenic nerves. This results in referred pain to either side of the neck or shoulders.
   — The spleen lies near the diaphragm and left phrenic nerve. This causes referred pain to the left neck and shoulder.
   — The liver lies beneath the diaphragm on the right. Inflammation and disease of the liver can result in referred pain along the phrenic nerve to the right neck and shoulder.
   — The heart and lungs lie superior to the diaphragm so epigastric pain is common. The stimulation of the vagal nerve may cause associated nausea and vomiting.
   — Appendicitis initially presents as visceral, poorly localized pain that may be peri-umbilical or epigastric.
   — Diverticulitis presents similar to appendicitis and often causes the same type of poorly localized pain in the epigastric/umbilical area.
   — Kidney stone pain is usually crampy or colicky and follows the ureter from the flank to the groin.

Slide 8-13

Areas of Referred Pain

▶ Review the locations of referred pain. Emphasize the importance of referred pain and the ability to predict organ involvement.

— Cholecystitis or gallbladder pain will be referred to the right scapulae or between the scapulae.

— The pancreas is located in the peritoneal and retroperitoneal space. It sits beneath the stomach and projects into the curve of the duodenum and the spleen. Because it is partially retroperitoneal, pain may be in the mid back.

— The abdominal aorta is a retroperitoneal structure. So pain from a tear in the aorta may produce visceral pain in the lumbosacral area with radiation to the anterior abdomen and legs.

— Bladder pain, because of its location, may be associated with low back pain.

— Pain associated with an AMI may refer to the arm, neck, jaw, or upper torso. This is because the visceral nerve fibers that supply the thoracic organs enter the spinal cord in the lower cervical and upper thoracic regions as do the parietal nerves fibers, once again making it difficult for the brain to localize the pain.

▶ Referred pain may be due to intra-abdominal or extra-abdominal causes.

Slide 8-14

Extra-Abdominal Causes of Pain

▶ Review the chart.

— An AMI may create diffuse abdominal pain and indigestion.

— Pneumonia may cause diffuse abdominal pain without local tenderness. Cough and fever may be present.

— In diabetic patients, elevated potassium may cause a squeezing sensation (like girdling) from the cramping of the smooth muscles.

— Drug withdrawal may present with severe colicky pain.

— Sickle cell disease patients may complain of severe abdominal pain due to splenic infarction.

— Spinal or CNS illness can cause chronic abdominal pain. The pain is often associated with inflammation of the spinal nerve roots (e.g., shingles).

▶ Remember that abdominal pain has many causes and you must focus on the patient, the presentation, and appropriate treatment, even if the exact cause of the pain is not identified.

Slide 8-15

What Is the Scene Telling You?

▶ Review the slide and emphasize that as part of your initial approach, you should complete a scene size-up and look for initial clues.

Slide 8-16

Characteristics of Blood in the Gastrointestinal Tract

▶ Review the types of bleeding and the significance of each.

— Hematemesis is associated with an upper GI bleed.

— Hematochezia is associated with a lower GI bleed. Blood is irritating to the GI tract and increases peristalsis causing diarrhea.

— Melena is a dark, black sticky stool. You often can differentiate melena from other causes of dark stool by the presence of diarrhea. Melena is often associated with diarrhea.

— Occult bleeding may not be visible in the stool if it is less than 100 cc. Chronic occult bleeding may lead to a hemoglobin loss and decrease the oxygen-carrying capacity of the blood.

Slide 8-17 **Initial Impression**
▶ Emphasize these factors in determining patient condition and for setting priorities.

Slide 8-18 **Focused History**
▶ Gather a history of the chief complaint by using the SAMPLE and OPQRST format. This can be done as treatment continues, or after transport is initiated.

Slide 8-19 **Factors That Affect Abdominal Pain**
▶ Emphasize that these factors affect the way patients perceive their pain.
— Children and infants may not be able to localize their pain so pay close attention to behavior and history.
— The obese and elderly tolerate pain better—potentially due to the presence of chronic pain or neuropathy.
— Pre-existing conditions such as the neuropathy of diabetes, alcohol, and medications such as steroids can mask abdominal pain.

Slide 8-20 **Factors That Affect Abdominal Pain (continued)**
▶ Patients do not perceive pain the same, so their perception of the pain severity may make the interpretation of the pain less reliable. Watch for patterns or progression. You may want to ask the patient to compare the pain to a different or previous pain incident to determine severity.
▶ The patient's mental state may affect pain perception. Hysteria coincides with an exaggeration of the pain. Emotional pain often worsens physical pain.

Slide 8-21 **Evaluate the Body Systems**
▶ As you are completing the assessment, it is often useful to review or clear each of the body systems. This is often useful when evaluating abdominal pain because so many of the body systems have components contained in the abdomen.

Slide 8-22 **Scenario 1 Scene Size-up**
Ask: *What does the scene suggest?*
— This appears to be a safe medical scene so far.
— No need for additional resources at this time.

Ask: *What is the patient telling you?*
— The patient is lying still with his knees drawn up suggesting parietal pain.
— He is in distress and not moving—possibly serious and need for early transport should be considered.

Slide 8-23 **Scenario 1 Initial Assessment**
▶ Initial assessment: Look for life threats and intervene if necessary.

▶ Initial impression:
— He is in distress.
— He does not appear to have
▪ an altered LOC.
▪ respiratory failure.
▪ deteriorating signs of shock.
▪ an immediate life threat.
▶ Paraphrase this information for the participants.
▶ When looking for an initial impression you can also ask:
— What may be wrong with this patient?
— What else could be wrong?
— Is this patient stable or unstable?
— What should be done next?
▶ This could be a GI bleed; ruptured bowel, appendix, or other structure; sepsis; sickle cell crisis; food poisoning; etc.
▶ Oxygen, IVs, and considering early transport may also be presented.

Slide 8-24 **Scenario 1 Focused Assessment and History**
▶ Allow participants to read the vital signs; then ask them if the vital signs support their initial impressions.

Ask: *What additional information is needed?*
▶ Acceptable responses:
— The vitals suggest a patient with hypertension, tachycardia, and tachypnea. His pulse oximetry suggests a need for oxygen.
— The vitals support the impression of distress.
— The high blood pressure and pale mucous membranes do not coincide.
— Additional information includes patient history to progress to the next slide that lists SAMPLE and OPQRST.

Slide 8-25 **Scenario 1 Focused History**
▶ Paraphrase this information for participants.
▶ Look for potential life threats and intervene if necessary.
▶ Review SAMPLE for any confirmation of their initial impressions:
S Symptoms suggests: gastrointestinal involvement
A Allergies suggests: none identified
M Medications suggest: possible GI irritation, cardiovascular considerations
P Past medical problems suggest: sickle cell disease, aortic aneurysm
L Last meal combined with symptoms suggest: food poisoning
E Events suggest: a new condition or sudden exacerbation of an existing condition
▶ Other: older black male with hypertension and nausea must be evaluated for an AMI

Ask: *What additional information needs to be obtained?*
— OPQRST and other appropriate questions.

Slide 8-26 **Scenario 1 Focused History**
- ▶ Paraphrase this information for participants.
- ▶ Look for potential life threats and intervene if necessary.
- ▶ Use the OPQRST to confirm the initial impression:
  - O Onset: The rapid onset confirms a sudden change which is an indication for early transport.
  - P Palliation/Provocation: The presentation confirms parietal pain.
  - Q Quality suggests solid organ pain. The pressure-like discomfort may suggest AMI pain. Because the pain is not crampy or colicky, the diagnoses of food poisoning or hollow organ involvement is decreased.
  - R Radiation: Pain goes into the back, which suggests cardiac pain, aortic pain, kidney pain, or pancreatic pain.
  - S Severity suggests an infarction. A severe pain indicates early transport.
  - T Time: The pain has stayed constant over time, which supports solid organ pain, or stretch pain from aortic involvement. Tends to eliminate food poisoning or bowel involvement.
- ▶ Additional information would include a physical exam and a review of systems to rule out problems.

Slide 8-27 **Scenario 1 Assessing Abdominal Pain**
- ▶ Emphasize looking for life threats.
- ▶ This could be a life threat.

Ask: *What are your differentials?*
- — Sickle cell crisis with splenic involvement is more likely, but pancreatic disease, aortic aneurysm, ruptured ulcer, and AMI, etc. are options to discuss.

Slide 8-28 **Scenario 1 Physical Exam**
Review and summarize.

Slide 8-29 **Scenario 1 Physical Exam**
Summarize.

Slide 8-30 **Scenario 1 Physical Exam**
Summarize.

Slide 8-31 **Scenario 1 Physical Exam**
Summarize.

Slide 8-32 **Scenario 1 Diagnosis: Sickle Cell Crisis with Splenic Infarct**
Autospleening usually occurs during childhood.

Slide 8-33 **Scenario 2 Scene Size-up**
- ▶ Answers reinforced:
  - — This appears to be a safe medical scene so far.
  - — No need for additional resources as yet.
  - — Recent dialysis, dizziness, and anticoagulant use are concerns.
  - — Concern about hepatitis due to dialysis history should also be considered.

Slide 8-34 **Scenario 2 Initial Assessment**
- ▶ Guide participants to look for life threats and intervene if necessary.

▶ Paraphrase this information for participants.

Ask: *What may be wrong with this patient? What else could be wrong? Is this patient stable or unstable? What should be done next?*

▶ This patient may be demonstrating early signs and symptoms of shock. Her airway is clear and her breathing is not compromised. Her mental status is adequate. Causes include dialysis, GI bleed, cardiac, or syncope.

▶ Participants should consider getting the patient in a supine position, initiating oxygen, IVs, and considering early transport.

▶ History, vital signs, and physical exam should be the next steps.

Slide 8-35 **Scenario 2 Vital Signs**

▶ Question if the vital signs support initial impressions. Ask what additional information they need.

▶ Acceptable responses:
  — The low blood pressure and pale mucous membranes correlate with GI bleeding or anemia.
  — A blood glucose of 90 for her could be significant; correlate it with her normal blood glucose.
  — BP in right arm due to AV-shunt.
  — Shock with GI bleeding, sepsis, bleeding somewhere else, electrolyte imbalance, etc.
  — The low pulse oximetry may be due to bleeding or anemia.

▶ This patient is showing early signs of shock. A tilt test is probably not indicated and may worsen her condition. The risk does not outweigh the benefit in this setting. If the participants opt for a tilt test, the patient would become dizzy as soon as they tried to help her sit up or stand. Allow participants to read the vital signs.

Slide 8-36 **Tilt-test**

▶ Review the slide. Point out that as in the scenario, if the patient becomes dizzy or loses consciousness, the test is positive and should be stopped.

Slide 8-37 **Scenario 2 Focused History**

▶ Paraphrase this information for participants.

▶ Look for potential life threats and intervene if necessary.

Ask: *Any confirmation of their initial impressions?*

▶ Then ask: What additional information needs to be obtained?
  S Her symptoms of feeling weak and dizzy suggest hypoperfusion or a syncopal episode, which is consistent with the initial impression.
  A None
  M Her medications suggest a significant medical history and should contribute to additional discussion of differential diagnoses.
    — Nitroglycerin for occasional angina suggests a cardiovascular problem.
    — Tenormin is a beta 1 adrenergic blocking agent and is used for its antianginal effects and antihypertensive effects. Tenormin may also prevent the heart from

increasing the rate in response to a hypotensive state. Tenormin is also associated with hypotension when given after dialysis.

— Potassium and lasix suggest a possible fluid and electrolyte imbalance.

— Erythropoietin is administered to renal failure patients because the kidney is no longer able to synthesize erythropoietin. Erythropoietin stimulates the production of red blood cells from the bone marrow. Without erythropoietin anemia results, which could contribute to her dizziness.

— Insulin indicates she is a diabetic and needs to be evaluated for her blood sugar because hypoglycemia may be a problem as well.

P Receives dialysis two times per week and is a diabetic, which support hypoglycemia and fluid and electrolyte imbalance. She is on anticoagulants, so occult bleeding may be a problem as well.

L Ate a light lunch 2 hours ago—her sugar should still be evaluated.

E Supports possible hypovolemia and/or electrolyte imbalance. The time suggests a new problem or sudden change of an old problem.

Slide 8-38 **Scenario 2 Focused History**

▶ Paraphrase this information for paticipants.

▶ Look for potential life threats and intervene if necessary.

Ask: *Any confirmation of your initial impressions?*

▶ Discuss the length of time she has had jelly stools and the implication.

O Indicates a recent change, or an inability to compensate.

P Exercise worsens the condition. Being still and sitting eases the condition, which reinforces hypoperfusion or a cardiac condition.

Q Denies pain.

R Denies pain.

S No complaint of pain.

T 20 minutes ago.

▶ Other: Because she is a diabetic and dialysis patient, she may have neuropathy and may not sense pain well.

Slide 8-39 **Scenario 2 Focused History**

▶ Neurological—The Cincinnati Stroke Test was indicated because she has several risk factors for a stroke and suffered a possible syncopal episode. Absence of neurological deficits tends to rule out stroke, but a TIA is still a possibility.

▶ Respiratory—Because she is not demonstrating any respiratory problems, the respiratory system involvement is not likely.

Slide 8-40 **Scenario 2 Focused Assessment**

▶ Her diabetic history, gender, and age may contribute to a non-classic presentation, so AMI should be considered, but

NOTES	SLIDE NO.	SLIDE TITLE/NOTES

aspirin and nitro are probably not indicated due to her history of heparin and hypotension.

Slide 8-41   **Scenario 2 Focused Assessment**
- ▶ Gastrointestinal—No, due to heparin use with dialysis, she could have occult blood loss.
- ▶ Renal—Because she was dialyzed today, fluid and electrolyte imbalances are possible.

Slide 8-42   **Scenario 2 Focused Assessment**
- ▶ Vascular—She may not compensate well to changes in pressure due to tenormin. GI bleeding is highly likely, but other causes of hypovolemia cannot be ruled out. Sepsis should also be a consideration.
- ▶ Consider her normal blood sugar. Many diabetics maintain a higher blood sugar as normal, so hypoglycemia may be a problem even though the readings are within the normal range.

Slide 8-43   **Scenario 2 Field Impression and Differential Diagnosis**
Review and summarize.

Slide 8-44   **Scenario 2 Gastrointestinal Bleeding**
Summarize.

Slide 8-45   **Scenario 2 Treatment of Gastrointestinal Bleeding**
Review the treatment. End of Scenario 2.

Slide 8-46   **Scenario 3 Scene Size-up**
- ▶ Paraphrase the information on the slide. Then ask . . .

Ask: *What does the scene suggest? What does the patient presentation suggest?*
- — This appears to be a safe medical scene so far.
- — No need for additional resources as yet. Syncope and early signs of shock are a concern.

Slide 8-47   **Scenario 3 Focused History**
- ▶ Paraphrase this information for the participants.

Ask: *What is your initial impression? What should be done next?*
- ▶ Acceptable answers:
  - — This patient's vital signs are within normal limits.
  - — This could be a GI bleed.
  - — This could be the flu.
  - — She may have an ectopic pregnancy or ovarian cyst.
  - — She has not eaten and her blood sugar should be checked.
- ▶ Factors to consider:
  - — Tubal ligation puts her at greater risk for ectopic pregnancy.
  - — Because she is a marathon bicyclist, her vital signs may suggest a problem because her normal pulse is 50–54.

Slide 8-48   **Scenario 3 Focused History**
- ▶ Paraphrase this information for the participants.

Ask: *Does this information change or support your initial impression? What else could be wrong?*
- ▶ Acceptable answers:

— The patient is showing early signs and symptoms of shock.

— The focused history supports the previous impressions.

▶ Factors to consider:

— Cramping indicates a hollow structure or organ involvement.

— Lower abdominal pain in women must include evaluation for reproductive system diseases and problems.

— Dizziness on standing indicates possibility of shock from hypovolemia.

— LLQ cramps indicate ovary, fallopian tube, colon, or ureteral.

Slide 8-49   **Scenario 3 Focused History**

▶ Paraphrase this information for participants.

Ask: *Does the information confirm or eliminate a diagnosis?*

▶ Acceptable answers:

— This patient is showing signs and symptoms of shock and is able to compensate as long as she is flat, which indicates a need for early transport.

— A GI bleed is less likely.

— The flu is still a possibility.

— She may have an ectopic pregnancy, ovarian cyst, or pelvic inflammatory disease (PID).

▶ Factors to consider:

— Dizziness on standing indicates possibility of shock from hypovolemia.

— LLQ cramps indicate appendix, ovary, or fallopian tube.

— Tubal ligations have a high correlation to ectopic pregnancies.

— Late period and sexually active point in the direction of possible pregnancy.

Slide 8-50   **Scenario 3 Follow-up**

▶ Review treatment.

— Rapid transport is indicated.

— Fluid replacement has improved her heart rate and was appropriate.

▶ When ovary/fallopian tubes rupture, they cause referred pain due to capsules rupturing and the chemical irritation from inflammation on the peritoneal lining, diaphragm, and phrenic nerves. This results in referred pain to either side of the neck or shoulders.

Slide 8-51   **Scenario 3 Follow-up**
Review. End of Scenario 3.

Slide 8-52   **Important to Note**
Remind participants that even though this lecture focused on identifying individual causes of acute abdominal pain, it is still essential to identify life threats and transport. They should not waste valuable time obtaining an in-depth field assessment on a critical or potentially critical patient.

Slide 8-53   **Summary**
Ask for questions and summarize.

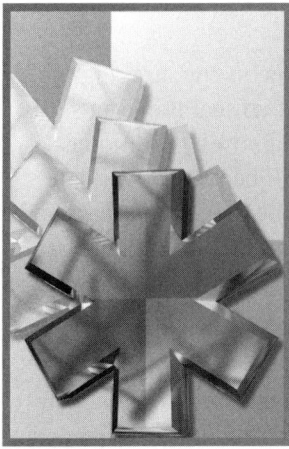

VI. ADVANCED MEDICAL LIFE SUPPORT INSTRUCTOR COURSE SLIDE NOTES

SLIDE NO.	SLIDE TITLE/NOTES
Slide I-1	**AMLS Instructor Course** Welcome and introductions as appropriate.
Slide I-2	**AMLS Instructor Course Objectives** Review the objectives.
Slide I-3	**AMLS Instructor Objectives** Review the objectives.
Slide I-4	**Instructor Prerequisites** Review the requirements to become an AMLS instructor. Emphasize the need for extensive anatomy, physiology, and pathophysiology knowledge and the ability to help the students sort through the processes.
Slide I-5	**AMLS Text and Course** The course and text are authored by separate groups. Each of the authors of the text possesses a wealth of knowledge and experience in emergency medicine and healthcare education. The AMLS course is designed and authored by the National Association of EMTs AMLS Committee. The National Association of EMS Physicians support medical guidance for the course.
Slide I-6	**Course Design** The course uses scenarios to relate the presenting symptoms to various diagnoses and how anatomy, physiology, and pathophysiology are associated with the symptoms. The scenarios are designed to build and refine the participants' experiences with medical emergency patients and guide them through the process of making a field diagnosis.
Slide I-7	**AMLS Focus** In order to identify a diagnosis, the participants will need to focus their assessment to refine the field diagnoses with the patient's presentation. As an instructor, you will present lectures and scenarios on patient assessment, dyspnea, chest discomfort, hypoperfusion, acute abdomen, and altered mental status.

NOTES

Slide I-8   **Diagnostic Model**
Review the slide contents with emphasis on encouraging the participants to use their assessment and critical thinking skills to form initial impressions and field diagnoses. Additional assessment and history-taking skills will be used to validate their diagnoses. These same skills will be used to reassess and confirm the management or care choices the participants have made are appropriate for the patient. Emphasize that knowledge of pathophysiology is a primary factor in using this process.

Slide I-9   **Process**
This type of model requires participants to form and validate links or connections from an assessment finding to a diagnosis. Using scenarios helps the students link between book knowledge and the patient conditions they encounter. Participants may have experiences, but need guidance to help with the links. You as the instructors will need to help with the experiences and guidance.

Slide I-10   **AMLS Goal**
Review

Slide I-11   **AMLS Course Philosophy**
Review

Slide I-12   **Diagnostic Model (Field Thinking Process)**
To form an initial impression, the participants will need to use the scene, patient affect or presentation, history, initial impression, and the mechanism of injury or nature of illness.

Slide I-13   **Diagnostic Model (Field Thinking Process)**
Review the slide. As the participants in the Provider course move through these steps, it is important for the instructor to continuously ask them to justify their answers. This will help reinforce the linking process and help identify valid and faulty reasoning.

Slide I-14   **Diagnostic Model (Field Thinking Process)**
Review the slide. The key is the use of information to validate the diagnoses or treatment modality they have chosen is an appropriate choice.

Slide I-15   **Diagnostic Model (Field Thinking Process)**
Review. Emphasize that with some settings, they will have a readily identifiable diagnosis. In other situations, they may not be able to come to one diagnosis, and will have to manage the symptoms.
The key is to assess and treat the patient and not get caught up into needing to have an absolute diagnosis each time.

Slide I-16   **Diagnostic Model (Field Thinking Process)**
Focus on reassessment during the management stage.

Slide I-17   **Diagnostic Model (Field Thinking Process)**
Review and summarize.

Slide I-18   **From Novice to Expert – The Dreyfus Model**
Describes the levels of expertise and how individuals operate within these levels.

Slide I-19 **The Novice**
- ▶ Entry-level.
- ▶ Has extensive book knowledge, but needs hands-on experience.
- ▶ Someone who has a good education can enter the workforce at the advanced beginner stage.

Slide I-20 **The Advanced Beginner**
- ▶ Has enough experience to be able to piece some blocks of information together but still has difficulty distinguishing between relevant and irrelevant information. (Is still a list follower.)
- ▶ This is usually the level one finds in the graduate paramedic or nurse, especially if she/he comes from an education program in which numerous case scenarios are managed.

Slide I-21 **The Competent Level**
- ▶ Can see the uniqueness of a situation—sees that it is not quite right, but still depends on the "rules" for dealing with a specific disease process and follows the set pattern.
  - — Is competent, but can't think outside the box. Is able to distinguish between relevant and irrelevant information during the healthcare process.

Slide I-22 **The Proficient Level**
- ▶ Able to gather blocks of information, weed out the irrelevant and the unique, and recall experiences from past events. Begins to see special situations earlier and with more experienced eyes.
- ▶ Sees the overall picture; has intuition.

Slide I-23 **The Expert Level**
- ▶ Able to recognize the patient in congestive heart failure by taking one look at the patient and without asking questions.
- ▶ Able to determine that a patient in the nursing home who has a sudden onset of shortness of breath accompanied by a cough as possibly having aspiration pneumonia and asks the right questions to rule it in.
- ▶ Often has correct "hunches" or gut feelings. This person would be a great mentor, as long as he/she can break down critical thinking skills for the learner.
- ▶ Uses analytic tools when a situation does not turn out as planned or when faced with a new situation.

NOTE: You may have six 3-person groups in your AMLS class comprised of 10 novices (students in a paramedic class) and eight experienced EMS providers who are at proficient and expert levels. How would you combine the groups?

Slide I-24 **Your Role as an Instructor**
Review.

Slide I-25 **Scenarios**
- ▶ Segue to a new discussion on how to conduct the group case scenarios.

Slide I-26 **Group Activity**
- ▶ Review how the practice and testing scenarios are chosen for each topic.

▶ Scenario 4 of each topic is used to test participants in the Provider and Refresher courses.

Slide I-27 **Group Activity**
▶ Instructors should read over each case assigned to them, organize the equipment, and prepare (moulage) the patient.
▶ Directions to the participants should include that a hands-on medical assessment and history-gathering will be expected, using AMLS principles. Each participant should take turns playing the role of team member and team leader as they practice—and test.

Slide I-28 **Group Activity**
▶ Have teams look over their equipment and go over last-minute instructions.
— The patient should assume the role described in the scenario and the instructor should read the scenario information.
— The first scenario of the course should be conducted slowly and allow for some interruptions. The remaining scenarios should be conducted as is.

Slide I-29 **The Initial Scenario Conducted for a Group**
▶ The first round of scenarios conducted for the assigned groups should be done in order to reinforce the principles of forming an initial impression with a list of differentials that can be ruled in and out.
▶ The instructor may let the group get started with its initial assessment—stop, and . . .

Ask: Is this patient stable or unstable?

Ask: *Should you go ahead and obtain a history or did your initial assessment indicate resuscitation is needed immediately? What's next?*
▶ After some assessment is completed . . .

Ask: *What is your field impression at this point?*
— Ask each team member.
▶ Compile the list of differentials or ask the group what its list should include.

Ask: *What should you do with this information? What's next?*
▶ Continue this format as participants compile information that leads toward a successful field impression with accompanying appropriate management.
▶ From this point on, the groups should perform as if they were on a real call—avoid input to the instructor other than answers to questions not answered through conversation with the prepared patient.

Slide I-30 **Initial Group Activity (continued)**
▶ Initial scenario, as described earlier. The field thinking process enforces critical thinking skills throughout the first round of scenarios.

Slide I-31   **Initial Group Activity (continued)**
▶ Reinforce that during the first group, rotations performed are step by step with instructor assistance; after that, allow the students to manage the scenario their way and make mistakes.

Slide I-32   **Group Activity**
The group may use their handouts (provided by NAEMT) as a reminder of the OPQRST and SAMPLE questions that should be asked.
▶ The instructor should provide positive reinforcement at the end of each case presentation and remind participants of the importance of good history-taking in order to form a correct field impression and effective management plan.

NOTE: If the team leader (especially a proficient or expert level provider) completed the scenario with a high level of success—quickly formed the correct field impression—have the leader review HOW he/she came to this correct impression. Guided review of this process is excellent for the novices or beginners in the group as well as the higher functioning providers.

Slide I-33   **Common Mistakes in Group Activity**
▶ Let the groups make these mistakes but review them upon summary.
▶ If a group leader incorrectly guides the participants through an incorrect field impression or differential diagnosis, the instructor should review the team's dynamics and AMLS assessment format.

Slide I-34   **Group Activity—Management**
▶ Critique upon completion of each scenario. Lead discussions with the group—do not lecture.
▶ Each diagnosis should be reviewed using appropriate anatomy and pathophysiology terminology.
▶ Instructors: Avoid tunnel vision. There is more than one way to do most things. Keep reinforcing the principles of AMLS—don't get bogged down on management.

Slide I-35   **Final Evaluation**
Review successful completion criteria.

Slide I-36   **Final Evaluation (continued)**
▶ Have the groups rotate through the final scenarios with each participant taking turns being team member and team leader.
▶ The instructor at each station must document each team's performance on the form provided.
▶ Scenario 4 is used for the final evaluation. Scenario 3 can be used for retesting. Remediate before retesting.

Slide I-37   **Course Coordination**

Slide I-38   **NAEMT**
▶ The National Association of EMTs sets the rules and administers the AMLS course, along with PHTLS.

▶ The National Association of EMS Physicians endorses this course and supports input for quality assurance of medical content.

Slide I-39 **The Coordinator & Instructor Guide**

▶ Slides and instructor notes within this Guide, along with the rules of course coordination, Differentiate between the set of slides purchased from Brady Publishing and those given to course coordinators and affiliate faculty from NAEMT.

— The current set of scenario-based lecture slide presentations and course administrative material is the 3rd edition.

— These new slides are from NAEMT for AMLS course coordinators and affiliate faculty.

Slide I-40 **Coordination of the Provider Course**

▶ This course cannot be conducted without providing the AMLS text to each participant and emphasizing the importance of reading it prior to the course. The cover letter, AMLS text, and pretest should be sent to the pre-registered participants at least one month in advance.

▶ This course is written for the advanced level EMS provider but can easily be used for flight nurses and emergency medicine nurses. For example, scenarios allude to the ED triage desk and the instructor must follow that format throughout the case for that team or team leader.

▶ BLS providers may challenge the course. They will be provided with a BLS pre-test and post-test. They will need to use the AMLS assessment and management philosophy throughout the course for successful completion.

Slide I-41 **The AMLS Refresher Course**

▶ The Refresher Course agenda is included in Part VII of this Guide.

▶ The agenda includes a review of initial impression and differential diagnoses within the patient assessment presentation and medical emergency case studies managed with moulaged victims.

Slide I-42 **AMLS Refresher Course**

▶ The 4-hour AMLS Refresher course is described as either an independent course or built within the second day of the Provider course.

— For those at the end of the 4-year certification period:

▶ Includes a 2-hour review of the five main topics of AMLS: hypoperfusion, dyspnea, chest discomfort and pain, altered mental status, and abdominal pain/GI bleeding with emphasis on the AMLS concept of medical patient assessment (i.e., use of initial impressions and differential diagnoses)

— There is one scenario per topic, with participant discussion integral to the review session.

— The instructor then reviews the pre-test with the participants.

— The participants are then organized into groups for evaluation rotations—Scenario 4 of each of the four main topics: dyspnea, chest discomfort and pain (which includes

shock), altered mental status, and abdominal pain/GI bleeding; along with the written exam.
— Successful completion allows another 4 years of AMLS certification.

Slide I-43   **AMLS Affiliate Faculty**
▶ Each international country and U.S. state will have at least one affiliate faculty, depending on geographic concerns and course activity.
▶ The role of the affiliate Faculty includes quality assurance and course administration for NAEMT.

Slide I-44   **Affiliate Faculty Qualifications**
▶ A listing of the affiliate faculty qualifications.
— Each applicant for affiliate faculty will be reviewed by the NAEMT AMLS Executive Committee.
— Experience in teaching, course administration, and quality assurance will be considered along with recommendations from AMLS Executive Committee members.
— Use the *AMLS Coordinator & Instructor Guide* for all the responsibilities and qualifications.

Slide I-45   **Course Coordinator Duties**
▶ The key to the success of an AMLS course is the local coordinator. This *AMLS Coordinator & Instructor Guide* provides guidance for the paperwork and rules of the course, but the coordinator needs to organize, advertise, and administer the course's daily operations. Upon course completion, the coordinator completes and sends the final course paperwork to the NAEMT office.
▶ We recommend that new instructors do not attempt to become course coordinators in their first AMLS course. Please ask for assistance from local course coordinators and affiliate faculty members.

Slide I-46   **Coordinator Qualifications**
Review information.

Slide I-47   **Job Description of the AMLS Course Coordinator**
Use the *AMLS Coordinator & Instructor Guide* for details in the qualifications and responsibilities of the course coordinators.

Slide I-48   **AMLS Instructor**
▶ Review the prerequisites for AMLS instructor.
— The affiliate faculty who monitors the new AMLS instructor will send a packet of information to the NAEMT office upon satisfaction of the requirements. This packet includes the two-sided AMLS Instructor Monitor form completed by the affiliate faculty.
— The AMLS instructor should teach at least one course per year.

Slide I-49   **Duties of the AMLS Instructor**
▶ The AMLS instructor must follow the rules of the NAEMT and the course authors who encourage inductive methods in case-based teaching and the development of critical thinking skills.

▸ During a course, instructors operate as a team and discuss how well the participants (as a whole and individually) are doing with the concepts and philosophy of the program.

▸ Experienced instructors should eventually be able to present several of the lectures within this program.

▸ Use the *AMLS Coordinator & Instructor Guide* for details on qualifications and responsibilities.

Slide I-50 **AMLS Medical Director Duties**

▸ The medical director: as charge of the medical content presented during the program, so has an integral duty in choosing who should present the information (i.e., faculty).

▸ Should always be available for any questions that may arise about the medical content or with administrative rules (along with the affiliate faculty).

Slide I-51 **AMLS Medical Director Qualifications/Duties**

▸ The medical director must: Be a licensed physician with an active interest in emergency medicine and with special knowledge in EMS. This is important because he/she is the resource person (along with affiliate faculty) for the course while adhering to NAEMT/AMLS course guidelines and standards.

▸ Use the *AMLS Coordinator & Instructor Guide* for details on the responsibilities and qualifications.

Slide I-52 **Participant Prerequisites**

▸ This course is written for the advanced level EMS or emergency medicine healthcare provider which presumes experience and knowledge in anatomy, physiology, and pathophysiology.

▸ Many training programs use this course format, adapt the agenda, and include it toward the end of their National Standard DOT Paramedic curriculum. It is used to summarize the medical emergencies sections and provides a forum for critical thinking skills labs in a scenario format.

▸ Basic level participants can receive a course completion certificate but need to take the basic level final written exam.

Slide I-53 **AMLS Course Coordination**

Review the participant-to-instructor ratio.

▸ There should be one instructor for every five participants for each scenario. There should be one instructor for every 2–3 participants for the final exam rotations.

Slide I-54 **Course Schedule**

▸ Some minor adaptations of the agenda can be done once the initial assessment and airway lectures are completed, but the lecture must precede the scenarios for each topic. Any deviation from the prescribed agenda must be approved in writing by the AMLS chairperson and NAEMT.

▸ The affiliate faculty and medical director should be made aware of any changes in the agenda.

Slide I-55 **Course Paperwork and Coordination**

▸ Refer to Section III in this Guide for the course application and budget forms.

— A course application and proposed agenda with faculty assignments should be sent to the NAEMT office (and affiliate faculty) 60 days prior to the course via the designated web-based software.

— The NAEMT office will send out a course packet that includes pre-test, post-test, and answer keys/reference sheets, certificates, handouts, and cards prior to the course. These will be mailed to the course coordinator.

— There will be some handouts for participants that may be used for math in drug calculations. The packet also includes a reference handout for SAMPLE and OPQRST history-gathering in the initial assessment.

▶ The NAEMT office will also send an invoice with the National Course Number assigned. The regional/state coordinator may assign the State Course Number.

▶ Each participant should complete the information requested on the application found at the back of this Guide.

▶ The NAEMT surcharge fee is $15 per participant for the Provider course, $10 per participant for the Refresher course, and $10 per participant for the Instructor course. All military courses are $10 per participant. Surcharge fees should be sent to NAEMT with course paperwork within 1 week following the course.

▶ Use the *AMLS Coordinator & Instructor Guide* for details on course coordination.

Slide I-56 **Continuing Education for AMLS**
▶ If no local EMS continuing education underwriter is available to the course coordinator, contact the CECBEMS. Currently, NAEMT assumes the responsibility of the cost of this resource.

▶ Most states approve this program for continuing education for nurses as well.

▶ The coordinator should investigate whether this program could be assigned college credit through the college of his or her choice.

Slide I-57 **Participant Packet**
▶ Review the participant packet (discussed earlier, along with the importance of reading the AMLS textbook).

Slide I-58 **Questions?**
Any questions?

Slide I-59 **Summary**
Summarize.

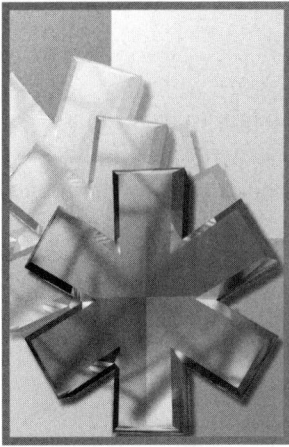

VII. REFRESHER COURSE SLIDE NOTES

⊞ ADVANCED MEDICAL LIFE SUPPORT

SLIDE NO.	SLIDE TITLE/NOTES

Slide R-1 **NAEMT**
Sponsored by the National Association of EMTs, this is a four hour program designed for those participants who completed the Advanced Medical Life Support (AMLS) Provider course within the last four years.

Slide R-2 **AMLS Refresher Review**
The first two hours of this program are designed to review the medical patient assessment via scenarios. We will then review the pre-test, the testing of scenarios, and the written exam.

Slide R-3 **Objectives**
Paraphrase the objectives of this initial session for the AMLS Refresher course.

Slide R-4 **Components of Assessment**
▶ The components of the medical patient assessment are staged into five essential steps with many secondary components within the steps.
▶ Decide whether this is a medical or a trauma call based on both the dispatch information and as part of the scene size-up. With confusing situations, the ability to determine whether the case is medical or trauma may have to wait until the focused history and physical exam.
▶ Identify and manage any immediate life threats in the initial assessment. This, along with the scene size-up, helps you determine whether this patient is stable or unstable and whether you should proceed to aggressive resuscitation or have time to perform a focused history and physical exam.
▶ Gather a patient history and perform a physical exam that is centered around the patient's chief complaint, even if unconsciousness is that complaint.
▶ Perform a detailed physical exam with vital signs.
▶ Provide continued and advanced medical care based on your differential impressions and continuously monitor the patient's condition with assessment of whether your treatment was effective. Communicate and document this information.

Slide R-5   **Scene Size-up**
- ▶ Based on the dispatch information, begin to develop a mental list of possibilities as to what's wrong with the patient. This continues as you approach and enter the scene. Scene size-up is the initial evaluation of the scene and the patient within it.
  - — What body substance precautions should I take?
  - — What hazards (or potential hazards) may be present?
    - ▪ Ensure safety of self, partner, patient, and bystanders.
  - — What other resources do I need to call for in this scene?
    - ▪ Is this a medical or trauma patient?
- ▶ The scene size-up should be continuously re-evaluated.

Slide R-6   **Initial Assessment**
- ▶ Recaps what has been done so far in our medical patient assessment.
- ▶ Prioritization and initial management are completed before we move on to gaining a history and performing a detailed physical assessment.
- ▶ In some patient situations, immediate transport may also need to be done.

Slide R-7   **Stable/Unstable**
- ▶ Is this patient physiologically stable or unstable? Often categorized by the seasoned EMS provider subconsciously: "Sick or not sick?"
- ▶ Stable means no immediate life threats. Unstable means that the patient is in need of immediate intervention, possibly early transport.
- ▶ This question is usually answered through assessment of the initial ABCD.
- ▶ Patient must be continuously reassessed.
- ▶ Look for the "red flags" of instability during the initial assessment.

Slide R-8   **Instability**
- ▶ Airway: Any sounds or signs of airway obstruction are key signs of instability.
- ▶ This would warrant immediate interventions prior to moving on to any other portion of the assessment.

Slide R-9   **Instability**
- ▶ Breathing: The general rate and work of breathing are assessed for "sick or not sick."
- ▶ Any accessory muscle use, poor air movement, irregular patterns, or extremes in rate (bradypnea or tachypnea) are all signs that the patient needs immediate interventions.

Slide R-10   **Instability**
- ▶ Circulation: Key indicators of instability within the circulatory assessment include these criteria.

▶ The assessment must include checking peripheral and central pulses, as well as skin vitals.

Slide R-11 **Instability**
▶ CNS: A sense of low Glasgow Coma score, with emphasis on the AVPU, and no spontaneous movement or inability to move extremities to command.

Slide R-12 **History**
▶ The OPQRST format guides the provider in gathering a thorough history of the chief complaint.
▶ It is centered on the complaint of pain or discomfort but can certainly be used for a dyspnea scale in those patients who are chronically or intermittently short of breath.

NOTE: If the patient indicates that his dyspnea is a high number on the scale, the provider should ask what happened the last time the patient's feelings of dyspnea were this severe (e.g., intubation, hospitalization).

Slide R-13 **Associated Complaints**
▶ Associated complaints are derived through direct questions. For instance, with a chief complaint of chest pain, the provider should ask direct questions as to whether the patient is having difficulty breathing, nausea, weakness, lightheadedness, or palpitations.
▶ If the patient denies these associated complaints, they are communicated and documented as pertinent negatives.

Slide R-14 **SAMPLE**
▶ Gain information on the patient's past medical history with use of the SAMPLE mnemonic. This helps you remember the pertinent questions.
▶ Make sure to ask about over-the-counter (OTC) medications as well as prescribed medications.
  — OTC medications include herbs and supplements.
▶ Obtain surgical and hospitalization history.

Slide R-15 **Unresponsive History**
▶ When the patient is unable to provide a history due to altered mental status, this becomes the chief complaint. AMS makes it even more imperative to gain clues from the environment. This patient is also considered unstable.

Slide R-16 **Focused Physical Exam**
▶ Perform a focused physical exam that is specific to the chief complaint.
  — Thorough head-to-toe assessment for unconscious patients.
▶ DO NOT develop tunnel vision while forming your initial impression.
  — EXAMPLE: I'm sure this patient who is having abdominal pain has cholecystitis, so I'm only going to examine the abdomen.

	SLIDE NO.	SLIDE TITLE/NOTES

Slide R-17

Ongoing Assessment

▶ A physical assessment is a continuous process. The ongoing assessment is completed after the focused history, physical exam, and initial management techniques.

▶ Re-evaluation is completed at routine intervals, based on the stability of the patient's condition.

▶ A final impression may not be formed until more diagnostic studies are completed in a definitive area of the hospital.

Slide R-18

Initial Impression

▶ The AMLS process of forming an initial impression . . .
— What could be wrong with this patient? (initial impression)
— What else could be wrong? (differential diagnoses)

▶ The process of forming the initial impression is based on the steps of the AMLS patient assessment.

▶ Experience on the part of the provider, an open attitude, and team collaboration are helpful in this process.

▶ Develop a treatment plan and re-evaluate whether the patient is getting better or worse and whether your initial impression needs to be revised.

▶ The process described is from the beginning to end of the call but the process continues into retrospective call review and continuing education within quality improvement activities.

NOTE: Segue into Scenario 1. We're now going to review the process of AMLS assessment, forming an initial impression with discussion of the clues to ruling in or ruling out the differentials of "What is wrong with this patient?"

Slide R-19

Scenario 1 Post-Operative Problems

NOTE: Teach the participants how these cases will be presented throughout this program. Audience participation is a must. Slides won't be advanced until the entire audience gets involved in answering questions and discussing procedures.

Slide R-20

Scenario 1 Scene Size-up

▶ Paraphrase the information on the slide. (DO NOT READ TO THE PARTICIPANTS.)

Ask: *Does this scene appear safe? Does this appear to be a medical or a trauma patient? From the doorway, does this patient appear to be stable or unstable?*
— Reinforce answers: This appears to be a safe medical scene so far. There appears to be a need for additional resources because the patient is heavy and there are some obstacles. Any patient with acute altered mental status is considered unstable.

NOTE: DO NOT advance to the next slide until the participants provide potential answers. Provide positive feedback for all responses and guide correct ones.

Slide R-21

Scenario 1 Initial Assessment

▶ Look for life threats and intervene if necessary.

▶ Paraphrase this information.

Ask: *What may be wrong with this patient? What else could be wrong? Possibilities?*
— Reinforce answers: This patient has an altered mental status. The possibilities include hypoglycemia, seizure, stroke, tumor, or any metabolic or structural problems in the central nervous system.

NOTE: DO NOT move to next slide until this slide has been discussed BY THE PARTICIPANTS!

Slide R-22   **Altered Mental Status**
▶ Paraphrase the OPQRST history with the Refresher group. Review the basics to the complications of gastric bypass procedures, including: aspiration, metabolic anomalies, post-operative infection, bowel obstruction embolus, and those complications of obesity.

Slide R-23   **SAMPLE History**
Review the SAMPLE history and encourage discussion.

Slide R-24   **Scenario 1**
▶ The initial treatment and diagnostics are seen on this slide. Ask the Refresher group what they should do with this information. Do not proceed until the group discusses this case.

Slide R-25   **Scenario 1**
This is a transition slide that begins to introduce the different causes of altered mental status. Ask for input from the group prior to advancing the slide. Encourage discussion.

Slide R-26   **Differentials for Altered Mental Status**
▶ Remember to look for the system that may be causing the altered mental status. We already know that this patient is hypoglycemic. We have ruled out arrhythmia. What should we do for this patient now?

Slide R-27   **Scenario 1**
▶ Paraphrase this information for the group regarding the failed attempt to correct the altered mental status by correcting glucose. With the added neurological signs, what differential diagnoses should we consider? Encourage discussion.

Slide R-28   **Altered Mental Status Differentials**
▶ A review of findings through the patient's history might give you a clue for the cause of the altered mental status. We see no signs of undiagnosed diabetes but this patient does have nystagmus.

Slide R-29   **Scenario 1 Differentials**
▶ Signs from the scene may give you a hint about the cause of the altered mental status. The patient's history does include an unusual nutritional state of late.

Slide R-30   **Altered Mental Status Differentials**
▶ The husband has reported this as bizarre behavior with confusion. As we take a look at some differentials we should consider, plus her recent weight loss and surgery, can we shorten our list of differentials?

Slide R-31 — **Differentials in Altered Mental Status**

▶ As we look at these potential causes for this condition, the instructor should point out that the patient is also exhibiting ataxic walking. What common differentials have we found thus far?

Slide R-32 — **Scenario 1 Differentials**

▶ Sometimes a complaint of pain will direct us towards a cause of altered mental status.

Slide R-33 — **Altered Mental Status Differentials**

▶ Has this patient's exam revealed any skin vitals that might warrant further investigation?

Slide R-34 — **Altered Mental Status Differentials**

▶ We've already determined that our patient in Scenario 1 does not have lateralizing signs. What quick neurologic exam might help here? Discussion should lead to either the Cincinnati Pre-Hospital Stroke Scale or the Los Angeles Stroke Scale.

Slide R-35 — **Scenario 1 Differentials**

▶ Our scene has revealed no signs of possible overdose but this review is a reminder not to overlook these clues.

Slide R-36 — **Altered Mental Status Differentials**

▶ Breathing patterns and breath odor can sometimes add information to our assessment. So far in Scenario 1, we haven't detected any change here.

Slide R-37 — **Scenario 1 Treatment**

▶ Hopefully by this time, the group has at least mentioned Wernicke's as a possibility. Please discuss the crucial role of thiamine in cellular glucose metbolism and why our dextrose administration failed to improve this patient.

Slide R-38 — **Scenario 1 Final Impression**

▶ Final impression, as discussed above with differentials.

ADD: Please discuss the pathophysiology and treatment of Wernicke's Encephalopathy. Refer to the current AMLS manual for supporting information.

Slide R-39 — **Scenario 2**
Title slide for Scenario 2

Slide R-40 — **Scenario 2 Shortness of Breath**

▶ Paraphrase the information on the slide in an attempt to paint the picture of the scene for scene size-up.

Ask: *Any concerns about this scene? Any resources needed at this time?*
— Reinforce answers: This does not appear to be an unsafe situation although the patient's complaint, along with his presentation as pale, may be of concern.

NOTE: DO NOT switch to the next slide until the group has discussed these questions with appropriate guidance and encouragement.

Slide R-41 **Scenario 2 Shortness of Breath**
▶ Review this information as the participants read it.

Ask: *Is this patient stable or unstable?*
▶ Begin the discussion around the cause of this patient's dyspnea and encourage the discourse on the differentials. Point out the patient's hypotension, tachycardia, chest wall pain, and pale skin. Segue to the next slide by asking the group to differentiate respiratory distress vs. respiratory failure.

Slide R-42 **Looking for Potential Respiratory Failure**
▶ Paraphrase the listed signs and symptoms as you ask whether this patient has potential respiratory failure. Segue to the next slide by pointing out that we need more information.

Slide R-43 **Finding the Cause of Dyspnea**
▶ In the OPQRST history gathering, some key findings in dyspnea include whether the symptoms came on suddenly or gradually.

Slide R-44 **History in Dyspnea**
▶ Additionally, use the severity scale to judge the patient's impression of how short of breath he/she is. This is useful for patients who have previous history of shortness of breath (COPD, asthma) for them to compare it to.

Slide R-45 **History in Dyspnea**
▶ Paraphrase the OPQRST history as noted on the slide. Ask the group whether they think this bizarre behavior may be related to our chief complaint—possibly hypoxia. As the group if the pleuritic chest discomfort rules out cardiac causes. Encourage discussion as to what additional information they require.

Slide R-46 **Scenario 2 SAMPLE History**
▶ Discuss the SAMPLE history and then ask about the patient's shock signs and symptoms—what could be wrong with this patient when pleuritic chest pain is combined with shortness of breath and there are shock signs? Encourage and support discussion.

Slide R-47 **Signs of Shock**
▶ The instructor/facilitator should review the differences in the various types of shock compared with our understanding of classic hypovolemic shock. This slide denotes non-hemorrhagic hypovolemic shock and how it may differ from "classic" shock. Segue to the next slide by asking what might cause obstructive shock.

Slide R-48 **Obstructive Shock**
▶ This slide confirms the three conditions that the group should have included as causes of obstructive shock. The instructor should discuss the pathophysiology of this type of shock.

Slide R-49   **Pulmonary Embolus Signs and Symptoms**
▶ This slide shows how pulmonary embolus signs and symptoms differ from our knowledge of classic shock. Ask the question from the slide on the risk factors for development of pulmonary embolus and whether the patient in Scenario 2 might have this condition.

Slide R-50   **Cardiac Tamponade**
This slide points out how cardiac tamponade presentation would differ from classic shock. Our patient has shock signs—but does he have signs of tamponade?

Slide R-51   **Tension Pneumothorax**
And finally, this condition of obstructive shock—tension pneumothorax, shows how the shock differs from the classic form. Do we need additional information to rule this condition in or out?

Slide R-52   **Distributive Shock**
Another form of shock is distributive. These are some of the conditions that cause this type. The instructor should discuss the pathophysiology of this type of shock and its effect on the vessels. The instructor should ask if the patient might have any of these conditions—and which one, with supportive discussion.

Slide R-53   **Scenario 2**
Back to Scenario 2—the instructor should remind the students of the case presentation to date (tachypneic, tachycardic, hypotensive patient with potential respiratory failure who complains of chest wall pain). Add a synopsis of the information on this slide and point out that the patient's psychiatric history might explain the presentation of bizarre behavior. Encourage discussion about what the impression should be with this additional information.

Slide R-54   **Scenario 2 Summary**
This is the summary slide for Scenario 2. Discuss the pathophysiology and treatment for this patient's hemopneuthorax from the earlier fall. Yes, this is a trauma case in a medical course, but remember, we should rule out trauma very early in our assessment of the patient. It was difficult with this patient due to his flight of ideas.

Slide R-55   **Scenario 3**
This is the title slide for Scenario 3: "He Can't Walk." Instructor segues to the next case.

Slide R-56   **Scenario 3**
Paraphrase the scene size-up for the participants while stimulating discussion with the question noted on the bottom of the slide.

Slide R-57   **Scenario 3**
The initial assessment should be reviewed with (not read by the instructor) the group with the questions asked. The instructor

might point out that there is an appearance of shock, except for the heart rate and blood pressure.

Slide R-58 **Scenario 3**
Some of the history obtained reveals a complaint of weakness with rectal pressure. The instructor should ask the group to differentiate potential causes of this presentation.

Slide R-59 **Scenario 3**
The SAMPLE history reveals a diabetic patient with cardiovascular disease and acute onset of unusual symptoms. Ask the group if there are any other possible causes.

Slide R-60 **Scenario 3**
A focused assessment reveals no obvious abdominal signs but complaints of continued rectal pressure. Could this be referred pain? The instructor should remind the group that diabetics have a hard time localizing pain due to their disease process. Let's review the potential causes of abdominal pain and referred pain.

Slide R-61 **Scenario 3**
The instructor should review the designated areas of referred pain with potential pathology (from the Abdominal [9] and GI [10] chapters of the current AMLS manual).

Slide R-62 **Scenario 3**
Areas of referred pain and potential causes continued from the back side.

Slide R-63 **Extra-Abdominal Causes of Abdominal Pain**
▶ The extra-abdominal causes of abdominal pain are listed by symptoms and differential diagnoses. This slide is also intended to pinpoint the cause of abdominal pain in Scenario 3.
— AMI may create diffuse abdominal pain and indigestion perceived as pain.
— Pneumonia may lead to diffuse abdominal pain with no local tenderness but cough and fever accompany the complaint.
— DKA: With high K+ levels, abdominal smooth muscles may cramp.
— Drug withdrawal creates a severe colicky pain.
— Sickle cell disease may cause severe abdominal pain due to splenic infarction.
— Spinal or CNS illness can cause pain referred to the abdomen.

Slide R-64 **Right Hypochondriac**
▶ Liver: steady, dull with radiation to right neck and shoulder from hepatitis, cirrhosis, with resulting ascites that may cause dyspnea or an distended abdomen.
▶ Gallbladder: tucked under the right lobe of the liver, typical right-upper quadrant pain with referral to right scapula or between the scapulae if stones.
▶ Referred pain to this area can come from pleuritis or pneumonia.

SLIDE NO.	SLIDE TITLE/NOTES

Slide R-65 **Epigastric**
- ▸ Stomach: located primarily in the epigastric region with possibilities of referred pain into left or right hypochondriac regions from gastritis.
- ▸ Pancreas: a 20-cm long organ behind the stomach that extends from the duodenum to the spleen; epigastric pain, bores into the back (retro).
- ▸ Referred pain to the epigastric region comes from AMI or appendicitis.

Slide R-66 **Left Hypochondriac**
- ▸ Spleen: located on the left behind the stomach and beneath the diaphragm; creates steady and dull pain with referral to the left shoulder and neck.
- ▸ Pancreas: as described in the previous slide; next to the spleen.
- ▸ Referred pain to this area is usually from pleuritis or pneumonia.

Slide R-67 **Central Abdomen**
- ▸ Small intestine: intermittent, crampy or colicky dull pain.
- ▸ Large intestine: from just beneath the stomach/liver and frames the small bowel.
- ▸ Aorta: a retroperitoneal organ that creates visceral pain in lumbar-sacral back/abdomen.
- ▸ Referred pain to this region is usually due to a large bowel obstruction.

Slide R-68 **Lumbar**
- ▸ Kidneys/ureters: Kidneys are located in the retroperitoneal space with dull and steady pain on posterior affected side. Ureters create colicky pain that many times refers to the groin.

Slide R-69 **Right Iliac**
- ▸ Appendix: Early inflammation can create periumbilical or epigastric pain but as it progresses, localizes to McBurney's point.
- ▸ Ovaries/fallopian tubes: Dull, constant pain in affected side is typical of ovarian problems. Fallopian tube pain is colicky and intermittent on affected side.

Slide R-70 **Left Iliac**
- ▸ Large intestine: as described earlier, mostly referred to the umbilical or hypogastric region.
- ▸ Left ovary and tube: as described in the previous slide.

NOTE: Recap Scenario 3: Middle-aged gentleman who thinks of himself as healthy developed epigastric pain with dyspnea two days ago. His abdomen exam is negative. Apparently newly diagnosed diabetes. In the ED with oxygen, IV, and a cardiac monitor on. Diagnostics being performed. Attempting to find the cause of his complaints.

Segue into next slide by reminding the group of the patient's presentation: rectal pressure and a feeling of weakness in a relatively stable patient.

Slide R-71 **Scenario 3 Update**
The instructor should allow the group to read this information with the summary statements. This has now become a very unstable patient. What would you like to do to—first stabilize the patient, then find out the potential causes.

Slide R-72 **Scenario 3**
The instructor should paraphrase the information as the students read it. Then ask the questions—promote discussion.
— Why (in presumptive hypovolemic shock) is the heart rate only in the 80s? (Discussion should include use of rate-controlled medication.)
— Differential diagnoses discussion should include retroperitoneal pathophysiology, such as abdominal aortic aneurysm, AMI (feeling of weakness and history), and diabetic complications.
— Additional treatment options might include bedside glucose, repeat ECG, advanced airway management, and transport with possible vasopressor drug delivery.

Slide R-73 **Scenario 3**
The local physician in charge of this case has given orders as listed. The instructor may discuss administration of dopamine in this setting.
If no response to the fluids AND the potential for distributive shock, a vasoactive agent may be indicated.

Slide R-74 **Scenario 3**
This slide includes updated patient information as the discussion of this case comes to an end. The patient's BP has rebounded and the group should discuss discontinuation (tapering) of the dopamine. This patient has an abdominal aortic aneurysm and his leg weakness is explained by aortic circulation to the spinal cord. The syncopal event and continued signs of poor perfusion are due to dissection of the aneurysm.

Slide R-75 **Scenario 4 Chest Pain Title Slide**

Slide R-76 **Scenario 4**
The instructor should summarize the background social information, along with the scene size-up information, then ask the questions with facilitated discussion of a potentially unstable patient.

Slide R-77 **Scenario 4 Chest Pain**
The instructor should summarize the information as a young, hypotensive patient with an irregular rhythm and a complaint of chest pain. Discussion as to treatment should be facilitated.

Slide R-78 **Scenario 4 Chest Pain**
As monitors are being applied, what other diagnostics and treatment should be provided? This is where the instructor can lead a discussion on the importance of treating this patient as if he's having an MI with 12-lead, IV, aspirin, and nitrates (if BP allows).

| | SLIDE NO. | SLIDE TITLE/NOTES |

The doubt in this will lie in the fact that the patient is so young. Can young people have heart ailments?

Slide R-79 **Scenario 4**
The instructor summarizes the history on the slide and facilitates discussion.

Slide R-80 **Scenario 4**
The instructor should summarize and facilitate discussion regarding a young male with an unusual presentation of syncope then left-sided chest pain with hypotension. Differentials might include AMI, trauma, spontaneous pneumothorax, or obstructive shock from PE. Slides 83 through 93 will assist the instructor in facilitating the discussion.

Slide R-81 **Scenario 4**
This slide adds more social history that confounds the situation. It points out that this patient may have an undiagnosed congenital disorder, along with other acute pathology.

Slide R-82 **Scenario 4**
This is a segue slide for the instructor to help guide discussion as to different causes of chest pain.

Slide R-83 **Chest Pain**
AMI
► AMI should be suspected in males over 30 and females over 40, especially with positive risk factors for this disease.
► Review classic signs and symptoms and then highlight that diabetics and females sometimes present without chest pain.
► Associated symptoms highlighted:
  — Physical findings are usually not helpful in the diagnosis.
  — An early 12-lead ECG needs to be done but not relied upon as THE diagnostic in identification of AMI, because a normal ECG can be seen in many ischemic cascades.
  — Standard treatment includes oxygen, IV fluids, and monitor(s), with aspirin early, and vasopressors for hypotension and pain management.

Slide R-84 **Aortic Dissection**
► Aortic dissection is fairly rare and hard to differentiate in the prehospital setting. The classic patient is a hypertensive male of 40–70 years of age.
► A tear in the intimal layer of the artery creates an artificial ballooning of the vessel (aneurysm) with pain that reflects the pathophysiology—tearing pain that is severe at first, then becomes intermittent. Depending on location of the dissection, symptoms vary:
  — Aortic arch: Carotid and subclavian involvement creates stroke-like symptoms or a pulseless arm. If it is extensive, it creates cardiac tamponade.

— Descending thoracic/abdominal/iliac aorta: These dissections traverse into the arteries that perfuse individual organs at times. For instance, iliac dissection may progress to the renal artery and symptoms might include hematuria.

▶ Depending on the location and symptoms, treatment may be either medical or surgical.

▶ Ehlers-Danlos syndrome: Inherited disorder of connective tissue that makes the vessels fragile. Aortic dissection may occur in younger patients with this disorder.

▶ Marfan's syndrome: Hereditary disorder of connective tissue that creates a tall, lean body with long extremities (fingers and toes). Aorta is dilated and susceptible to dissection.

Slide R-85   **Pulmonary Embolism**

▶ Pulmonary embolism (discussed in earlier case as obstructive shock) may produce chest pain. If more than half of the pulmonary vasculature is involved, this is a serious, life-threatening condition with shock symptoms, dyspnea, and hypoxia.

▶ Symptoms may be described as sharp, pleuritic chest pain, tachycardia, and tachypnea. Physical findings not usually helpful but lung sounds may include crackles and pleural rub.

▶ Discuss the risk factors associated with 80% of PEs.

Slide R-86   **Esophageal**

▶ Perforation of the esophagus occurs with sudden, forceful rise in the intra-abdominal or intrathoracic pressures (e.g., forceful vomiting, coughing, or post-procedures such as endoscopic exam).

▶ GI contents leak into the mediastinum—overwhelming infection will occur, but chest pain is first. Chest pain is sharp, steady in the anterior, posterior, and epigastric regions. May radiate to the neck. Associated symptoms include dysphagia and hemoptysis with pleural friction rub, tachycardia, tachypnea, and hypotension.

▶ Esophageal perforation occurring in the hospital is usually due to medical instrumentation of para esophageal surgery. Medical procedures cause over one-half of all perforations and can be caused by any instrument that enters the esophagus. Out-of-hospital perforations are either traumatic or spontaneous. Spontaneous perforation most commonly results from a sudden increase in intra-esophageal pressure, combined with negative intra-thoracic pressure, which is caused by straining or vomiting. Other causes include: caustic ingestion, Barrett's ulcer, and infectious ulcers in patients with AIDS and following dilation of the esophageal strictures.

▶ Treatment is geared to supporting the septic patient with monitors, oxygen, fluids, and transport to a cardiothoracic surgeon.

Slide R-87   **Cardiac Tamponade**

▶ Cardiac tamponade develops in a medical setting via the accumulation of fluids into the pericardial sac. This fills to

the point of compromising cardiac filling and drops cardiac output—thus shock.
— If from an infectious condition like pericarditis, chest pain may be present.

▶ Malignant pericardial effusion does not usually present with chest pain, but may have symptoms similar to pericarditis (positional chest pain). Renal failure patients who accumulate fluid tend to create pericardial and pleural effusions without pain.

▶ If tamponade, Beck's Triad may be apparent.

Slide R-88 **Tension Pneumothorax**

▶ Tension pneumothorax, as a cause of chest pain, has been discussed earlier in the obstructive shock portion of this review.

▶ Tension pneumothorax in a medical setting usually occurs with congenital or acquired weakened thoracic tissue, creating a simple pneumothorax that progresses. This can also occur in COPD patients, those with cancer of lung tissue, or lung infections.
— This phenomenon occurs with much more frequency during positive pressure ventilation, especially with co-existing lung disease.

▶ If chest pain occurs, it is sudden and sharp, pleuritic in nature, and accompanied by tachypnea, dyspnea, and tachycardia, with splinted respirations.

Slide R-89 **Pericarditis**

▶ An inflammatory condition that produces steady, burning, retrosternal chest pain that may radiate into the back, neck, scapula, or jaw. It may worsen with deep breath and pulsate with each beat of the heart. It is worse upon lying down— improves with sitting up or leaning forward (positional chest pain).

▶ A pericardial rub might be heard if conditions were silent in the environment and the healthcare provider was trained to auscultate this abnormal heart sound. There may be ST-segment elevation or PR depression in many leads, without localization.

Slide R-90 **Costochrondritis**

▶ Inflammation of the ribs and cartilage supporting the ribs may develop after an upper respiratory infection. The chest pain is usually sharp and made worse by chest wall and arm movement.

▶ There may be point tenderness at the site upon palpation of the chest wall. But patients suffering from AMI and PE may also have point tenderness, so costochondritis should never be diagnosed in the field.

Slide R-91 **Pleurodynia**

▶ Inflammatory condition of the parietal pleura with sharp, pleuritic pain and few other symptoms

▶ No or few physical findings, possibly a pleural friction rub; similar to costochondritis.

Slide R-92 **GI Disorders**
- ▸ GI disorders can cause chest pain, too.
- ▸ Peptic ulcer disease (PUD), acute cholecystitis, esophagitis, esophageal spasm, and gastroesophageal reflux (GERD) are some conditions that may cause this.
  - — Sensory nerve fibers are shared between many abdominal structures and the thorax.
- ▸ Usually retrosternal burning, similar to AMI. May radiate to the throat and cause heartburn. Worse at night, especially when lying supine or leaning far forward.
- ▸ Esophageal spasm is just like an AMI in appearance and usually improves with administration of nitroglycerin. (Conversely, AMI pain can be relieved with antacids.)

Slide R-93 **Mitral Valve Prolapse**
- ▸ Elastic mitral valve expands into the left atrium during systole and can create episodes of chest pain due to stretching of the chordae tendinae and papillary muscles.
- ▸ Associated symptoms include vertigo, dyspnea, palpitations, and syncope.
- ▸ Systolic murmur (click) and cardiac dysrhythmias may be found. Most patients with this condition are asymptomatic.

Slide R-94 **Scenario 4**
The physical exam of our patient is described. The instructor should describe scoliosis and pectus excavatum (congenital "funnel breast"), and the systolic click. Point out the appearance of a patient with Marfan's Syndrome (without revealing it). Marfan's is an inherited disorder of connective tissue affecting the musculoskeletal and cardiovascular systems. Manifests in young adulthood with tall, gangly limbs, arachnodactyly (spider fingers), and kyphoscoliosis.

Slide R-95 **Scenario 4 Summary**
This is a summary slide for the instructor to point out a mitral valve prolapse and/or mitral regurgitation. The instructor could go back in the slide sequence to slide 93 to review signs and symptoms. Remind the group that most mitral valve issues have no signs nor symptoms. The mitral valve bulges its leaflets into the left atrium at systole. The syndrome of mitral valve prolapse includes a systolic click, left chest pain, and fatigue with syncope and dyspnea. The symptoms may include hypotension, palpitations, and orthostasis.

Slide R-96 **Scenario 5**
Title slide.

Slide R-97 **Scenario 5**
The instructor should paraphrase the scene size-up for this patient, and discussion should ensue about respiratory precautions against infectious diseases—specifically droplet spread and good handwashing.

SLIDE NO.	SLIDE TITLE/NOTES
Slide R-98	**Scenario 5** The instructor can paraphrase and describe a patient in obvious respiratory distress. The group should easily identify this as unstable. Signs and symptoms of varicella may be discussed. A discussion on differentiating respiratory distress from failure would be good (repeat from earlier discussion).
Slide R-99	**Scenario 5** Review the initial assessment of this ill patient and ask the group for initial treatment and any diagnostics or information needed.
Slide R-100	**Scenario 5** The instructor should paraphrase the history thus far and ask for an initial impression and differential diagnoses thus far. The patient seems alert enough to be in respiratory distress with high potential for respiratory failure. Differentials might include ARDS, pneumonia, aspiration, Guillain-Barré syndrome with respiratory distress, or exacerbation of a pre-existing disease.
Slide R-101	**Scenario 5** The SAMPLE history adds some more information, and the instructor should facilitate a discussion on the field impression and list of differentials. The instructor can then segue into next slide, reminding the group of the different causes of dyspnea. Slides 102–107 will assist the instructor with the differentials (and previous discussion from Slide 100).
Slide R-102	**Scenario 5** Recapped by the instructor. Note that the patient had no history.
Slide R-103	**Scenario 5** Additional causes of dyspnea listed. Ask the group if these should be considered in our patient.
Slide R-104	**Scenario 5** The instructor may summarize more causes of dyspnea and facilitate ruling in/out these as causes.
Slide R-105	**Additional Causes of Dyspnea** Discussion.
Slide R-106	**Causes of Dyspnea** The instructor discusses neuromuscular diseases that may precipitate dyspnea.
Slide R-107	**Cause of Dyspnea** Discuss the last few causes listed for dyspnea and facilitate discussion as to their relevance in our case. The instructor can then introduce the next slide by reviewing the case thus far.
Slide R-108	**Focused Exam** Discuss the focused exam and some early treatment. The instructor should then ask the group the questions prior to the next slide.

Slide R-109   **Scenario 5**

The instructor should re-open the discussion of respiratory distress vs. respiratory failure as a topic opener for the possibility of intubation in this case. The discussion should then proceed to the special precautions to use with the infectious patient in an intubation attempt.

Slide R-110   **Scenario 5 Summary**

This is a summary slide for the instructor to wrap up Scneario 5, our last case. Additional information to add is that 20–30% of Varicella cases in adults go onto develop pneumonia and sepsis, especially in the elderly—many of whom succumb to this illness. Varicella has a 21-day incubation period and requires respiratory/droplet precautions, along with standard precautions.

Slide R-111   **Questions**

This has been intended to be a review of the five major AMLS topics: hypoperfusion, dyspnea, abdominal pain, chest pain, and altered mental status via a case study format. The course will proceed to review the pre-test questions, test the group/team on these five topics, and then give the written exam.